MUSCULAR SYSTEM - ANATOMY, FUNCTIONS AND INJURIES

MUSCULOSKELETAL DISEASES

TYPES, CAUSES AND TREATMENTS

MUSCULAR SYSTEM - ANATOMY, FUNCTIONS AND INJURIES

Additional books in this series can be found on Nova's website under the Series tab.

Additional e-books in this series can be found on Nova's website under the e-book tab.

MUSCULAR SYSTEM - ANATOMY, FUNCTIONS AND INJURIES

MUSCULOSKELETAL DISEASES

TYPES, CAUSES AND TREATMENTS

GREG REED
EDITOR

New York

Library of Congress Cataloging-in-Publication Data

ISBN: 978-1-63463-551-6

Library of Congress Control Number: 2014955558

Published by Nova Science Publishers, Inc. † New York

Contents

Preface

This book provides an analysis of costs of musculoskeletal disorders of employed individuals. It also discusses the application of differential scanning calorimetry for the diagnosis of musculoskeletal disorders, and the effects of stretching and sensory motor training for older adults with musculoskeletal disorders.

Chapter I – Musculoskeletal Disorders (MSD) are one of the leading classes of health effects and can be caused by various factors, work related and nonwork related. MSD refers to health related problems of the locomotor apparatus, i.e. health problems of the skeleton, ligament, muscles, tendons, joints, nerves and cartilage. Rates of MSD vary by population, their age groups, genders, socioeconomic aspects and other factors. These factors can affect the author's understanding of the prevalence, incidence, and costs of MSD aside from the variability of actual prevalence or incidence rates due to etiologic issues or costs due to illness or injury severity or treatment response and recovery. This chapter focuses on types of MSD of employed individuals, and associated medical costs and demographic factors. The US Bureau of Labor Statistics (BLS) classifies occupational MSD as cases where nature of injury or illness is pinched nerve; herniated disc; meniscus tear; sprains, strains, tears; hernia (traumatic and nontraumatic); pain, swelling, and numbness; carpal or tarsal tunnel syndrome; Raynaud's syndrome or phenomenon; musculoskeletal system and connective tissue diseases and disorders, when the event or exposure leading to the injury or illness is overexertion and bodily reaction, unspecified; overexertion involving outside sources; repetitive motion involving micro tasks; other and multiple exertions or bodily reactions; and rubbed, abraded, or jarred by vibration. The economic burden of occupational MSDs is very high. BLS reports that about 30 percent of all occupational injuries involving days away from work are due to MSDs.

While some studies have focused on economic burden, here the author's concentrate on the costs of assessment and treatment of MSDs. MarketScan databases are used to analyze these medical costs by ICD9 codes for the year 2010. These databases consist of millions of records on medical claims classified by ICD9 codes, different medical cost components and some socioeconomic and demographic variables. The results obtained in this study suggests that the average costs per person among the three body regions (neck, upper back and lower back) of focus in this analysis were found to be highest for upper back in the inpatient data and for lower back in the outpatient data. Approximately half (25 out of 47) ICD-9 codes with the highest average costs per person in the inpatient data consisted of intervertebral disc, spinal stenosis, and spinal curvature codes. Of the outpatient service records examined, 23 out of 50 codes were for intervertebral disc, spinal curvature, and spinal stenosis diagnoses.

Chapter II – Background: Despite of the improved biochemical analyzes and imaging technology, diagnosis of different types of musculoskeletal diseases is still challenging. New methods are needed to improve the diagnostic procedures and help to select the most sufficient treatment. Aims: The purpose of the author's current review was to demonstrate the usefulness of differential scanning calorimetry in the intraoperative diagnosis of musculoskeletal diseases. Materials and methods: Different types of ligaments, connective tissues, joint capsules, arthritic or septic hyaline cartilage were collected intra operatively from pathologic, or healthy human origin. The thermal denaturation of the samples was monitored by a SETARAM Micro DSC-II calorimeter. Results: Here the author's demonstrated a significant difference in the pattern of the thermal denaturation characteristics of the degenerative or inflamed collagen tissue samples, compared with the healthy human connective tissue. The degenerative samples' thermal enthalpy was significantly decreased, while the melting temperature showed an increase. In case of the inflamed samples, the author's found a significant increase in the enthalpy and a decrease of melting temperature. Conclusion: These data suggest that DSC analysis could be a clinically relevant, additional method in the intraoperative diagnosis of different types of musculoskeletal diseases.

Chapter III – The ageing process is responsible per se for a series of morphological and functional alterations of the musculoskeletal system, which can compromise the functional independence of the elderly. It is common the decrease in muscle mass (sarcopenia) and in muscle force (dinapenia). It also occurs increase in the stiffness of the muscle-tendon unit, decrease in fascicle length and in the pennation angle related to the aged. These changes negatively affect the muscle strength and may also impair the mobility, balance and gait of the older adults. When associated with physical inactivity there is a potentiation of the deleterious effects resulted from aging process, and these situations can be recognized as musculoskeletal diseases. Still, the poor mobility associated with decrease in muscle strength and balance can increase the chances of falls in this population. Thus, to mitigate and/or reverse these changes it has been recommended regular physical activity and//or systematic exercise. A number of different types of exercise have been suggested, among them stretching, neuromotor and balance exercises are emphasized. Stretching exercises, when performed by a period equal to or greater than four weeks with three to four repetitions and duration between 30 and 60 seconds, has proved to be effective not only in improving flexibility and range of motion, but also gait speed, which is related with a lower risk of falls. Among the neuromotor exercises, video game exercise training has been shown to be effective in improving balance, agility and muscular strength, and also in reducing the risk of falls in community elderly. For a specific balance training, it has been recommended that this must be composed by gradual exercise in complexity and support base, starting from simple postures and greater support and developing throughout training; dynamic movements that can alter the center of gravity, recruiting postural muscles; and can also reduce the sensory imput information, for example, perform the same exercise, but with eyes closed. The training should be performed two to three times a week, lasting 20-30 minutes per session. Thus, it is emphasized the importance of exercise for older people, especially regular stretching, balance and neuromotor ones can be adopted to prevent and/or improve flexibility, balance, mobility, comorbidities and musculoskeletal diseases in this population.

In: Musculoskeletal Diseases
Editor: Greg Reed
ISBN: 978-1-63463-551-6

Chapter I

Analysis of Costs of Musculoskeletal Disorders of Employed Individuals

Anasua Bhattacharya and Sudha P. Pandalai
Centers for Disease Control and Prevention,
National Institute for Occupational Safety and Health,
Cincinnati, US

Abstract

Musculoskeletal Disorders (MSD) are one of the leading classes of health effects and can be caused by various factors, work related and nonwork related. MSD refers to health related problems of the locomotor apparatus, i.e. health problems of the skeleton, ligament, muscles, tendons, joints, nerves and cartilage. Rates of MSD vary by population, their age groups, genders, socioeconomic aspects and other factors. These factors can affect our understanding of the prevalence, incidence, and costs of MSD aside from the variability of actual prevalence or incidence rates due to etiologic issues or costs due to illness or injury severity or treatment response and recovery.

This chapter focuses on types of MSD of employed individuals, and associated medical costs and demographic factors. The US Bureau of Labor Statistics (BLS) classifies occupational MSD as cases where nature of injury or illness is pinched nerve; herniated disc; meniscus tear;

sprains, strains, tears; hernia (traumatic and nontraumatic); pain, swelling, and numbness; carpal or tarsal tunnel syndrome; Raynaud's syndrome or phenomenon; musculoskeletal system and connective tissue diseases and disorders, when the event or exposure leading to the injury or illness is overexertion and bodily reaction, unspecified; overexertion involving outside sources; repetitive motion involving micro tasks; other and multiple exertions or bodily reactions; and rubbed, abraded, or jarred by vibration

The economic burden of occupational MSDs is very high. BLS reports that about 30 percent of all occupational injuries involving days away from work are due to MSDs. While some studies have focused on economic burden, here we concentrate on the costs of assessment and treatment of MSDs. MarketScan databases are used to analyze these medical costs by ICD9 codes for the year 2010. These databases consist of millions of records on medical claims classified by ICD9 codes, different medical cost components and some socioeconomic and demographic variables.

The results obtained in this study suggests that the average costs per person among the three body regions (neck, upper back and lower back) of focus in this analysis were found to be highest for upper back in the inpatient data and for lower back in the outpatient data. Approximately half (25 out of 47) ICD-9 codes with the highest average costs per person in the inpatient data consisted of intervertebral disc, spinal stenosis, and spinal curvature codes. Of the outpatient service records examined, 23 out of 50 codes were for intervertebral disc, spinal curvature, and spinal stenosis diagnoses.

Introduction

Musculoskeletal Disorders (MSD) refers to health related problems of the locomotor apparatus. The World Health Organization defines MSD as health problems of the skeleton, ligament, muscles, tendons, joints, nerves and cartilage (Luttman, 2003). The US Bureau of Labor Statistics (BLS) classifies occupational MSD as cases where nature of injury or illness is pinched nerve; herniated disc; meniscus tear; sprains, strains, tears; hernia (traumatic and nontraumatic); pain, swelling, and numbness; carpal or tarsal tunnel syndrome; Raynaud's syndrome or phenomenon; musculoskeletal system and connective tissue diseases and disorders, when the event or exposure leading to the injury or illness is overexertion and bodily reaction, unspecified; overexertion involving outside sources; repetitive motion involving micro tasks; other and multiple exertions or bodily reactions; and rubbed, abraded, or jarred by vibration. MSD can be classified by International Statistical Classification of Diseases, ninth revision (ICD-9) codes, and also by the nature and anatomic location of injury or illness.

MSD, one of the largest class of health effects (Timpka et al., 2014; Woolf et al., 2012; Woolf et al., 2010; Freburger et al., 2009; Sinnott and Wagner, 2009; Brooks, 2006), is caused by various factors, work related and nonwork related, and rates of MSD vary by population, their age groups, genders and other factors. Prevalence rates have been reported ranging from 35% for upper back MSD among health care workers (Long et al., 2013), to 90.6% lifetime prevalence for any MSD among farmers (Osborne et al., 2012). Determination of such rates for MSD depend on a range of factors such as type of study used to assess rates (Driscoll, 2011), definition of outcome used to assess MSD (Saarni et al., 2007), or use of a diagnosis code or rating of function to characterize MSD cases for analysis of health impacts, costs, and other effects (Rudolf et al., 2012; Kostanjsek et al., 2010). These factors can affect our understanding of the prevalence, incidence, and costs of MSD aside from the variability of actual prevalence or incidence rates due to etiologic issues or costs due to illness or injury severity or treatment response and recovery. The ICD-9 diagnosis and procedure, Diagnosis-related group (DRG), Current Procedural Terminology (CPT), and the Healthcare Common Procedure Coding System (HCPCS) codes (CMS, 2014) have been used to examine patterns of illness and injury and their management and outcomes in various types of data, and to determine costs associated with MSD. These codes, predominantly ICD-9 codes, have been used to evaluate medical costs in administrative databases (Sears et al., 2013; Lix et al., 2012), but there are challenges to these efforts. Codes that accurately capture MSD diagnoses (Sinnott et al., 2012) or procedures (Clement et al., 2013) require appropriate selection and validation (Walvern and Austen, 2012; Walvern et al., 2011) to avoid bias and results that lead to incorrect association of treatments with diagnoses (Clement et al., 2013; Ensor et al., 2013) and incorrect assessment of health impact, resource utilization, and costs (Benchimol et al., 2011; De Coster et al., 2006).

The economic burden of occupational MSD is very high. BLS reports that about 34 percent (BLS, 2013) of all occupational injuries involving days away from work are due to MSD. According to the current global burden of disease study, MSD are the second most common cause of disability worldwide, measured by years lived with disability (YLDs), with low back pain being the most frequent condition (Vos, et al., 2012). The study also found that disability due to MSD is estimated to have increased by 45% from 1990 to 2010, in particular osteoarthritis, and is expected to continue to rise with an increasingly obese, sedentary and aging population. Earlier research on the global burden of occupational diseases and injuries found that the annual incidence of MSD represented 31% of all occupational diseases estimated in the world in 1994 (Leigh et al., 1995). Gardner *et al.,* (2008) identified MSD as the leading work-related health concern in the developed world, accounting for up to 30% of all injuries requiring time away from work. This study signifies that MSD are the most frequent occupational disease that affects workers throughout the world. The number of work-related diseases reported in Sweden in 2003 was 25,391 cases for employees and self-employed persons, with a rate of 61 cases per 10,000 workers. Swedish official statistics report that ergonomics factors (monotonous or unusually strenuous movements or work posture) were the cause of 58.5% of all work-related diseases with a rate of 35.7 cases per 10,000 workers (Sveriges Official Statistics, report 2005). Finland found 4,807 occupational diseases in 2002 (20 cases per 10,000 workers), out of which 28 percent were repetitive stress injuries (MSD caused by non-physiological stress in work such as repetitive and monotonous work, unusual working posture) with a rate of 5.7 cases per 10,000 workers. Diagnoses of specific repetitive stress injuries in Finland included mononeuropathy of upper and lower extremity, hand and arm vibration syndrome, epicondylitis, tenosynovitis, peritendinitis, and bursitis, among others (Riihimaki, et al., 2004). In 2012, 905,690 injuries and illnesses that required recuperation away from work were reported in private industries in USA. During the same year, over 388,060 MSD (34%) were reported, accounting for more than one in three injuries and illnesses with days away from work (BLS, 2013).

The magnitude of economic losses associated with MSD depends on several factors, for example, the severity of the condition, the nature and quality of health care received, characteristics of the patient, such as age and general health status, and how the loss is measured. Conventionally, costs of occupational diseases are classified into direct costs and indirect costs (Leigh et al., 2000). However, non-health related factors, for example, psychosocial factors, workplace characteristics, and availability of disability compensation, are also important determinants of the economic losses associated with MSD (Baldwin, 2004). In addition, the socioeconomic factors of populations in different countries influence the results of the magnitude of MSD (Andersson, 1998).

Researchers estimated losses due to MSD to range from 0.5% to 2% of GDP (Blair et al., 2003). In separate cost analysis for specific MSD, low back pain (LBP) was found to be the most expensive MSD in the workplace. LBP causes the loss of 149 million workdays annually in USA (Guo et al., 1999). The cost of medical treatment for all work-related back pain was estimated as US $13 billion in 1990 with an estimated growth rate of 7% per year (Stratus, 2002). In 1992, back cases represented 24% of U.S. Workers' Compensation claims and 31% of the costs. The estimated cost of back problems between 1988 and 1992 in some states of the USA was US $8,244 per claim with 38% accounting for health-care cost, and 62% for indemnity costs (Williams et al., 1998). According to Gore et al., (2010) patients with chronic low back pain have greater comorbidity and economic burdens compared with those without chronic low back pain. This economic burden can be attributed to greater prescribing of pain-related medications and increased health resource utilization. According to Kartz (2006) total costs associated with low back pain in the United States exceed $100 billion per year, two-thirds of which are a result of lost wages and reduced productivity.

The median days away from work for MSD cases was 9 days in 2012, compared to 8 days in 2010 for all days away from work cases (BLS, 2011; BLS, 2013). According to the American Federation of Labor and Congress of Industrial Organizations (AFL-CIO) 2012 report 'Death on the Job, The Toll of Neglect: A National and State-By-State Profile of Worker Safety and Health In the United States', from 1992 through 2010, the percent of MSD were the highest in 2000 (35%) and total cases of MSD involving days away from work were the highest in 1992 (784,100) (AFL-CIO, 2012). The percent of MSD cases was 29.4 in 2008 and 2009 but increased to 30.5 percent in 2010 (AFL-CIO, 2012). The burden of MSD is not equally shared across the population. Sengupta et al., (2009) reported that the recovery time for musculoskeletal injuries increases significantly with age. Tanaka et al., (2001) estimated that about 40% of all upper extremity MSD in the US workforce was attributable to occupational exposures. There are also numerous studies estimating the costs of MSD in the United States (Webster and Snook, 1994, Brogmus et al., 1996, Hashemi et al., 1998, National Research Council and Institute of Medicine, 2001; Baldwin, 2004, Peele et al., 2005, Silverstein and Adams, 2007, the American Academy of Orthopedic Surgeons, 2008, and Dunning et al., 2010) and other countries (Woolf and Pfleger, 2003, and Piedrahita, 2006). Some of these studies include all MSD, some of them concentrate only on upper extremities, and others focus on some specific types of MSD. Most of these studies emphasize estimating direct costs of MSD. Bhattacharya (2014) evaluated research on direct and indirect costs of occupational MSD in the US and estimated the direct and indirect costs of occupational MSD and CTS for the years 2003 through 2007. This study found that the direct costs of MSD were $1.5 billion and the indirect costs were $1.1 billion for the year 2007. Webster and Snook (1994) reported an average compensable cost of $8,070 per case for 1989 for “upper extremity cumulative trauma disorder” claims from a large, national Workers' Compensation (WC) insurance carrier with coverage in 45 jurisdictions. The median cost was $824. Brogmus et al., (1996) found that work-related MSD of the upper extremity averaged $6,760 per claim for the year 1992. This average was 80% higher than the average of all claims ($3,723) reported to Liberty Mutual in 1992. According to 1995 estimates by the National Research Council and the Institute of Medicine (2001), annual direct costs of all MSD (occupational and non-occupational MSD) were $215 billion, whereas estimates for work-related MSD ranged between $45 and $54 billion for the year 1998. Morse et al., (1998) found that work-related MSD significantly reduced the ability of individuals to perform activities of daily living in Connecticut. Silverstein and Adams (2007, a technical report) reported that the direct costs of work-related MSD of neck, back and upper extremity were $6.8 billion and averaged $11,903 per case during the years 1997 through 2005 for the state of Washington. Dunning et al., (2010) utilized WC claims data from the Ohio Bureau of Workers' Compensation (OBWC) and found that the average total cost per claim was $5,130 (medical costs were $2,924 and indemnity costs were $,2206). The American Academy of Orthopedic Surgeons (2008), editor of ‘The Burden of Musculoskeletal Diseases in US’ (page 227), used data from the Medical Expenditure Panel Survey and stated that the US average per person cost of MSD for all population (both working and non-working populations) was $5,824 for the years 2002–2004. Most of the research described above has focused on costs of MSD and economic burden. This chapter focuses on types of MSD diagnosis in a dataset of employed individuals and associated medical costs and demographic factors. Several types of MSD are examined in this chapter.

Data and Methodology

Data

MarketScan databases are used to analyze medical costs by ICD-9 codes for the year 2010. These databases consist of millions of records on medical claims classified by ICD-9 codes, different medical cost components and some socioeconomic and demographic variables. This database is focused on healthcare costs and contains information on employees of participating employers including utilization of medical care, the industry they are employed in, their gender, age group, and region (a description of the MarketScan databases is available on request, Hansel and Chang, 2010 white papers). The data comprise inpatient, outpatient, and pharmacy services covered by group health insurance system for employed individuals aged zero to 64. MarketScan data specifies for each month in which an employee is enrolled for medical insurance the employee age, gender, type of health insurance coverage, region of the U.S., industrial sector, and employee status (hourly/salaried; union/non-union). Seven industrial sectors were represented: retail trade; transportation, communication and utilities; manufacturing durables; manufacturing non-durables; services; finance, insurance and real estate; and oil and gas extraction/mining. The regions included South, Northeast, North Central, West and "unknown." The data released by Thomson Reuters MarketScan to external clients has been certified as de-identified according to HIPAA rules. Due to these stringent confidentiality requirements, workers could not be classified by individual (identity-protected) employer.

The data used in this study consists of medical expenses of individuals classified by ICD-9 codes related to MSD, and the corresponding procedure codes, and DRG codes of the individuals that filed for these MSD related medical claims. Expenses related to these medical claims are estimated as the *total costs* including out-of-pocket expenses not covered by the insurance benefits. The group health medical expenditure can run from a nominal amount for individuals with few medical claims to very large numbers for those with numerous medical claims related to MSD. The distribution, therefore, is a normal distribution as the medical expenses are continuous in nature.

The data used here from MarketScan databases are comprised of medical claims classified by two primary categories, inpatient admissions and outpatient services for the year 2010. These medical claims were classified by different demographic variables and the final inpatient database had 18,209 employees that had filed for 29,250 medical claims related to MSD. The average cost for an MSD claim was $65,236.

Table 1a illustrates the descriptive statistics of the inpatient admission claims of the population studied here by their demographic variables. The sample had 53 percent females with most of them in the age group of 55 to 64 years employed mostly in the manufacturing, durable sector.

Table 1a. Demographics for Inpatient Admissions. Age, gender, and industry variables were assessed in the Medstat database as discussed in the methods

		Age groups					
Industry	Gender	0-17 years	18-34 years	35-44 years	45-55 years	55-64 years	Total
Oil, Gas and Mining	Male	8	19	28	53	41	149
	Female	10	27	36	68	35	176
Manufacturing, Durable	Male	63	117	311	598	562	1651
	Female	98	167	332	647	507	1751
Manufacturing, Nondurable	Male	33	86	200	319	232	870
	Female	69	87	208	322	189	875
Transportation, Communication, and Utilities	Male	44	148	288	414	340	1234
	Female	109	191	314	421	310	1345
Retail	Male	12	30	62	97	69	270
	Female	12	41	55	93	101	302
Finance, Insurance and Real Estate	Male	48	149	214	314	294	1019
	Female	79	204	257	355	230	1125
Services	Male	52	144	293	394	413	1296
	Female	90	267	318	489	480	1644
All	*Male*	348	876	1807	2846	2640	8517
	Female	*616*	*1,283*	*2,006*	*3,220*	*2,566*	*9,691*

The sample had the highest number of male population in the age group of 45 to 54 years of age, and most of them were employed in the manufacturing, durable sector. Most of the sample resided in the southern region (not noted in the table).

Table 1b illustrates the descriptive statistics of the outpatient services medical claims by their demographic variables. The final outpatient database had 2,053,331 employees that had filed for 5,896,443 medical claims related to MSD. The sample had 56 percent females with most of them in the age group of 45 to 54 years with the highest employment in the services sector. The sample had the highest number of male population in the age group of 45 to 54 years of age, and most of them were employed in the manufacturing, durable sector. Most of the sample resided in the southern region (not illustrated in the table).

Table 1b. Demographics for Outpatient Admissions. Age, gender, and industry variables were assessed in the Medstat database as discussed in the methods

		Age groups					
Industry	**Gender**	**0-17 years**	**18-34 years**	**35-44 years**	**45-54 years**	**55-64 years**	**All**
Oil, Gas and Mining	Male	771	2,637	3,353	5,569	4,172	16,502
Manufacturing, Durable	Male	9,563	19,279	32,520	58,231	40,554	160,147
	Female	15,724	20,445	36,212	63,901	41,032	177,314
Manufacturing, Nondurable	Male	5,015	11,108	20,375	27,150	17,769	81,417
	Female	9,439	11,671	20,018	30,415	16,391	87,934
Transportation, Communication and Utilities	Male	8,867	24,494	39,509	48,347	29,566	150,783
	Female	15,668	26,682	40,618	55,419	29,781	168,168
Retail Trade	Male	1,267	3,939	5,979	7,325	5,917	24,427
	Female	2,159	5,678	6,513	10,282	7,778	32,410
Finance, Insurance and Real estate	Male	7,174	21,246	28,024	28,840	20,951	106,235
	Female	13,102	25,422	32,006	37,204	24,143	131,877
Services	Male	13,944	29,628	39,531	44,145	37,003	164,251
	Female	20,797	49,913	54,118	66,761	50,102	241,691
All	Male	58,154	140,515	217,067	284,398	213,206	913,340
	Female	97,382	180,671	252,143	363,834	245,646	1,139,676

Methodology

ICD-9, DRG, and Procedure Codes

Selection of MSD related ICD-9 codes was based on codes suggested by a review of several studies that evaluated specific ICD-9 codes for neck, upper back, and lower back MSD (Sinnott et al., 2012). A list of 122 unique ICD-9 codes was identified for use in the present analysis. Codes related to fracture, pediatric or congenital diagnoses were excluded from this analysis. Codes related to dislocation were included since fracture-dislocation situations should have fracture coded as the diagnosis. The consideration of spinal curvature codes is supported by several reports in the literature. Increased lumbar spine stiffness was found to occur even after 1 hour (in men) or 2 hours (in women) of continuously working on office work tasks in a sitting posture (Beach et al., 2005). Concurrent decreases in low back pain and improvement in thoracic kyphosis and lumbar lordosis (as measured biomechanically) have been observed in nurses participating in a spine training program (Jaromi et al., 2012). An earlier study found an association between a diagnosis of scoliosis and report of chronic low back pain in the preceding year in nurses (Violante et al., 2004). A study of oyster shuckers, who have among their occupational exposures standing for long periods of time in awkward postures, with sustained neck and back flexion, were found to have higher levels of kyphosis than the general population (Hsu et al., 2011). In light of such information, codes related to spinal curvature (scoliosis, kyphosis, and lordosis) from Sinnott and colleagues (2012) were included in this analysis. A full listing of this starting pool of ICD-9 codes is available upon request from the authors.

Formulation of Body Region Variables

Body region designations for ICD-9 codes were assigned based on whether the diagnosis was nonspecific, neck (cervical), upper back (thoracic), or lower back (lumbar). The non-specific category includes codes that relate to "not otherwise specified" designations, multiple site diagnoses, or codes that for one reason or another do not specify a body region. Diagnoses that related to both the thoracic and lumbar regions were included in the lumbar region category. The number of codes in each group was as follows: nonspecific=39, neck (cervical) =39, upper back (thoracic) =14 and lower back (lumbar) =30.

Data Extraction and Analyses

Records were extracted from the data that had a medical claim related to one of the 122 ICD-9 codes of neck, upper back, or lower back MSD. Costs were analyzed for body region, and data for the top ICD-9, DRG, and CPT codes were examined with further descriptive analyses. Multinomial logistic regression analysis was conducted to examine the costs for different body regions. Statistical analyses were conducted using Stata and SAS (Stata, 2013; SAS, 2010). The body parts were used as the dependent variable. The different demographic variables and logarithm of total costs of each individual for the different medical claims were used as the independent variables.

Results

Analysis of costs examined average cost per person by body regions and demographic variables. These costs were analyzed using medical claims data on inpatient admissions and outpatient services (Table 2). The overall average costs per person by body region was $63,055 (inpatient)/$253 (outpatient) for neck, $89,500/$288 for upper back, and $55,537/$380 for lower back, whereas the non-specific diagnoses had the highest average cost for inpatient admissions at $105,489 and lowest for outpatient services at $246. Costs for inpatient admissions exceed outpatient care by a factor of 200 or more.

Analysis of average costs per person for individual ICD-9 codes is presented in Tables 3a and 3b. Analysis of inpatient admissions (Table 3a) revealed that while the highest cost was for code 839.21 (closed dislocation of thoracic vertebra), the average costs for the top fifteen diagnoses ranged from $111,650 to $257,645. In these fifteen codes, six codes were related to spinal curvature diagnoses, one code was related to intervertebral disc disease in the thoracic region, one code was related to spondylosis (unspecified), and the remainder were related to dislocation of vertebra at various cervical and thoracic levels. Forty-seven of the top fifty codes (20 of these codes are represented in Table 3a and the rest are in Appendix A) with the highest average cost had an N greater than 2. Among these, 9,748 individuals had a diagnosis of intervertebral disc related disorders (12 ICD-9 codes), 4,869 individuals had diagnoses related to spinal stenosis codes (2 codes), and 2,431 had diagnoses related to spinal curvature diagnoses (11 codes).

Other code related groups included those related to vertebral dislocations (N=120), spondylosis with or without myelopathy (N=276), and postlaminectomy syndromes (N=469). The diagnosis of other, pain disorder related to psychological factors occurred for 1,478 individuals with an inpatient average cost per person of $36,411.

Among outpatient records (Table 3b), the highest average cost is for ICD-9 code 737.21, lordosis postlaminectomy, with an average cost of $1,169 for 124 individuals in the dataset.

Table 2a. Percentage Distribution of Demographic Variables and Average Costs by Body Region for the Inpatient Admissions

Body Region	Nonspecific			Neck (Cervical)	Upper Back (Thoracic)		Lower Back (Lumbar)		All
	Percentage (%)	Average Costs ($)	Percentage (%)	Average Costs ($)	Percentage (%)	Average Costs ($)	Percentage (%)	Average Costs ($)	Average Costs ($)
Females	11	99,868	5	59,111	2	77,684	35	55,926	65,739
Males	5	117,419	5	67,387	2	103,027	35	55,146	64,662
0-17	4.5	7,847	0.18	127,177	0.1	87,160	0.52	54,039	111,372
18-34	2.81	65,059	0.67	49,626	0.47	92,628	7.91	45,091	51,945
35-44	1.83	67,386	2.34	56,242	0.59	57,778	16.17	51,889	53,900
45-54	3	118,255	4.44	59,969	1.17	85,351	24.7	57,178	64,046
55-64	3.5	131,044	2.77	72,811	0.92	113,819	21.4	60,303	71,897
Oil, Gas and Mining	0.32	83,422	0.37	54,178	0.05	62,411	1.63	55,473	59,203
Manufacturing, Durable	3.29	114,812	2.44	56,748	0.8	60,523	18.29	50,924	60,275
Manufacturing, Nondurable	1.71	95,783	1.33	53,762	0.43	120,399	9.27	50,118	58,993
Transportation, Communication and Utilities	3.22	119,801	1.82	60,146	0.66	91,653	13.12	56,870	69,175
Retail Trade	0.69	107,812	0.44	60,557	0.08	44,956	2.96	58,751	66,823
Finance, Insurance and Real estate	2.34	106,046	1.84	69,749	0.45	87,586	11.01	55,475	65,653
Services	3.61	94,092	2.25	55,971	0.71	70,943	14.87	52,057	60,174
Northeast	1.83	119,000	1.21	57,804	0.37	87,664	8.49	48,801	61,710
North Central	3.67	92,435	1.88	58,673	0.82	73,019	17.11	51,698	59,378
South	6.1	103,833	4.85	56,382	1.3	85,485	29.02	56,467	64,368
West	3.98	114,706	2.43	82,520	0.76	115,198	15.95	61,704	74,772
Unknown	0.06	49,759	0.02	40,766			0.14	37,696	41,243
All	15.64	105,489	10.4	63,055	3.25	89,500	70.71	55,537	65,236

Table 2b. Percentage Distribution of Demographic Variables and Average Costs by Body Region for the Outpatient Services

Body Region	Nonspecific		Neck (Cervical)		Upper Back (Thoracic)		Lower Back (Lumbar)		All
	Percentage (%)	Average Costs ($)	Percentage (%)	Average Costs ($)	Average Costs ($)	Average Costs ($)	Percentage (%)	Average Costs ($)	Average Costs ($)
Females	7.98	244	6.12	257	3.8	294	37.62	372	335
Males	3.95	248	3.76	247	2.9	280	33.88	387	356
0-17	5.09	202	0.83	166	0.51	198	1.14	245	204
18-34	1.92	235	1.92	205	1.46	250	10.35	355	312
35-44	1.45	265	2.47	254	1.6	288	17.33	379	352
45-54	1.96	293	3.01	285	1.93	311	24.68	385	365
55-64	1.51	325	1.65	29	1.19	333	18	393	378
Oil, Gas and Mining	0.26	227	0.13	294	0.13	299	1.79	420	384
Manufacturing, Durable	2.44	228	2.05	230	1.15	295	15.95	380	344
Manufacturing, Nondurable	1.26	248	0.91	264	0.57	303	8.1	418	379
Transportation, Communication and Utilities	2.51	240	1.43	273	1.36	303	15.11	385	354
Retail Trade	0.42	235	0.26	248	0.19	318	2.78	374	346
Finance, Insurance and Real estate	2.16	247	1.12	231	0.83	305	11.13	385	350
Services	2.44	256	5.35		2.31	252	15.87	360	316
Northeast	1.85	228	0.84	253	0.64	329	8.64	387	350
North Central	2.44	258	5.36	227	2.47	244	18.34	351	310
South	4.84	248	2.12	314	1.97	311	30.74	376	354
West	2.75	243	1.55	259	1.6	309	13.62	420	373
Unknown	0.05	243	0.01	245	0.01	345	0.16	388	333
All	11.93	246	9.87	253	6.7	288	71.5	380	345

Tables 2a and 2b. Inpatient (2a) and Outpatient (2b) Average Costs by Body Regions and Demographic Variables: The table presents the costs for data evaluated from the Medstat database, as described in the methods, by body regions and demographic variables.

Table 3a. Average Costs by ICD-9 Codes, Body Regions– Inpatient Admissions

ICD-9	Diagnosis	Body Region	N	Minimum Cost	Maximum Cost	Average Cost
83921	Closed dislocation thoracic vertebra	Upper Back (Thoracic)	11	1,982	815,136	257,645
83906	Closed dislocation sixth cervical vertebra	Neck (Cervical)	27	2,800	960,585	196,000
73743	Scoliosis associated with other conditions	Nonspecific	102	2,200	1,009,265	195,855
73739	Other kyphosis and scoliosis	Nonspecific	297	2,200	1,767,411	194,381
83901	Closed dislocation first cervical vertebra	Neck (Cervical)	18	11,093	1,283,143	189,957
73740	Unspecified curvature of spine associated with other conditions	Nonspecific	7	7,328	642,250	182,631
83902	Closed dislocation second cervical vertebra	Neck (Cervical)	10	12,483	927,736	178,245
72272	Intervetebral disc disorder with myelopathy thoracic region	Upper Back (Thoracic)	61	6,844	1,677,783	168,960
83903	Closed dislocation third cervical vertebra	Neck (Cervical)	7	32,103	626,817	168,430
83908	Closed dislocation multiple cervical vertebrae	Neck (Cervical)	20	3,058	558,142	140,235
73729	Other lordosis acquired	Nonspecific	22	6,698	678,102	139,023
73719	Other kyphosis acquired	Nonspecific	49	1,592	326,183	124,555
72191	Spondylosis of unspecified site with myelopathy	Nonspecific	17	12,242	605,391	119,308
83905	Closed dislocation fifth vertebra	Neck (Cervical)	13	3,276	604,938	116,148
73734	Thoracogenic scoliosis	Upper Back (Thoracic)	30	12,016	450,791	111,650
73710	Kyphosis (acquired) (postural)	Nonspecific	201	1,120	770,125	110,989
83907	Closed dislocation seventh cervical vertebra	Neck (Cervical)	10	7,532	364,428	106,923

ICD-9	Diagnosis	Body Region	N	Minimum Cost	Maximum Cost	Average Cost
83904	Closed dislocation fourth cervical vertebra	Neck (Cervical)	15	10,932	536,216	101,938
73730	Scoliosis (and kyphoscoliosis) idopathic	Nonspecific	1671	-	2,060,064	99,468
72282	Postlaminectomy syndrome of thoracic region	Upper Back (Thoracic)	20	13,635	661,909	95,320

Table 3b. Average Costs by ICD-9 Codes, Body Regions– Outpatient Services

ICD-9	Diagnosis	Body Region	N	Minimum Cost	Maximum Cost	Average Cost
73721	Lordosis postlaminectomy	Nonspecific	124	0	7567.559	1169.701
72282	Postlaminectomy syndrome of the thoracic region	Upper Back (Thoracic)	1292	0	105699.6	944.4302
72232	Schmorl's nodes of lumbar region	Upper Back (Thoracic)	1267	0	13357.01	660.6234
72280	Postlaminectomy syndrome of unspecified region	Nonspecific	4216	0	123875.2	640.6244
72231	Schmorl'e nodes of thoracic region	Neck (Cervical)	673	0	10776.48	628.1806
73722	Other postsurgical lordosis	Nonspecific	33	0	5436.52	573.1309
72402	Spinal stenosis, lumbar region, without neurogenic claudication	Lower Back (Lumbar)	164655	0	576000	558.7106
72283	Postlaminectomy syndrome of lumbar region	Lower Back (Lumbar)	72333	0	228544.6	518.212
73712	Kyphosis postlaminectomy	Nonspecific	132	0	19500	502.5141
72292	Other and unspecified disc disorder of thoracic region	Upper Back (Thoracic)	2830	0	52424.78	444.057

Table 3b. (Continued)

ICD-9	Diagnosis	Body Region	N	Minimum Cost	Maximum Cost	Average Cost
72239	Schmorl's nodes of other spinal region	Nonspecific	109	0	6686.706	434.2996
72293	Other and unspecified disc disorder of lumbar region	Lower Back (Lumbar)	38030	0	135522.1	416.1764
72271	Intervetebral disc disorder with myelopathy cervical region	Neck (Cervical)	27277	0	182600	405.5709
83918	Open dislocation multiple cervical vertebrae	Neck (Cervical)	40	0	3808	402.4312
72210	Displacement of lumbar intervertebral disc without myelopathy	Lower Back (Lumbar)	509568	0	203999.9	396.5939
72141	Spondylosis with myelopathy thoracic region	Upper Back (Thoracic)	1924	0	54527.88	387.083
72211	Displacement of thoracic intervertebral disc without myelopathy	Upper Back (Thoracic)	25282	0	56989.05	380.8786
72401	Spinal stenosis of thoracic region	Upper Back (Thoracic)	4538	0	53898.26	368.6751
72291	Other and unspecified disc disorder of cervical region	Neck (Cervical)	19258	0	36727.03	364.2701
72272	Intervertebral disc disorder with myelopathy thoracic region	Upper Back (Thoracic)	2161	0	19262.66	357.8098

Legend: Tables 3a and 3b. Average Costs by ICD-9 Codes, Body Regions. The top 20 ICD-9 codes with the highest average costs per person are presented with inpatient data in Table 3a and outpatient data in Table 3b. The following 30 ICD-9 codes with the highest average costs per person are presented with inpatient data in Appendix A and outpatient data in Appendix B.

Table 4a. Average Costs and Number of People by DRGs, CPTs, ICD-9 Codes, Body Regions– Inpatient Admissions

DRG Codes		Procedure Codes		ICD-9 Codes	Diagnosis	Body Regions	N	Minimum Cost	Maximum Cost	Average Cost
454	Combined anterior/ posterior spinal fusion with CC	8105	Dorsal and dorsolumbar fusion of the posterior column, posterior technique	73730	Scoliosis (and kyphoscoliosis) idiopathic	Nonspecific	6	167,382	773,802	524,106
454	Combined anterior/ posterior spinal fusion with CC	8106	Lumbar and lumbosacral fusion of the anterior column, anterior technique	73730	Scoliosis (and kyphoscoliosis) idiopathic	Nonspecific	13	105,866	650,725	303,774
456	Spinal fusion except cervical with spinal curvature/malignancy/infection or extensive fusions with major complications and comorbidities	8105	Dorsal and dorsolumbar fusion of the posterior column, posterior technique	73739	Other kyphoscoliosis and scoliosis	Nonspecific	6	28,213	572,142	301,337
456	Spinal fusion except cervical with spinal curvature/malignancy/infection or extensive fusions with major complications and comorbidities	8105	Dorsal and dorsolumbar fusion of the posterior column, posterior technique	73739	Other kyphoscoliosis and scoliosis	Nonspecific	14	56,509	612,065	291,851
457	Spinal fusion except cervical with spinal curvature/malignancy/infection or extensive fusions with complications and comorbidities	8105	Dorsal and dorsolumbar fusion of the posterior column, posterior technique	73739	Other kyphoscoliosis and scoliosis	Nonspecific	15	36,856	714,039	289,008
456	Spinal fusion except cervical with spinal curvature/malignancy/infection or extensive fusions with major complications and comorbidities	8105	Dorsal and dorsolumbar fusion of the posterior column, posterior technique	73730	Scoliosis (and kyphoscoliosis) idiopathic	Nonspecific	40	29,872	1,264,711	269,420

Table 4a. (Continued)

DRG Codes		Procedure Codes		ICD-9 Codes	Diagnosis	Body Regions	N	Minimum Cost	Maximum Cost	Average Cost
457	Spinal fusion except cervical with spinal curvature/malignancy/infection or extensive fusions with complications and comorbidities	8105	Dorsal and dorsolumbar fusion of the posterior column, posterior technique	73739	Other kyphoscoliosis and scoliosis	Nonspecific	13	71,947	627,912	265,542
454	Combined anterior/ posterior spinal fusion with CC	8108	Lumbar and lumbosacral fusion of the anterior column, posterior technique	73730	Scoliosis (and kyphoscoliosis) idiopathic	Nonspecific	7	125,953	484,440	227,954
458	Spinal fusion except cervical with spinal curvature/malignancy/infection or extensive fusions without major complications and comorbidities	8108	Lumbar and lumbosacral fusion of the anterior column, posterior technique	73739	Other kyphoscoliosis and scoliosis	Nonspecific	6	47,567	591,330	227,687
454	Combined anterior/ posterior spinal fusion with CC	8106	Lumbar and lumbosacral fusion of the anterior column, anterior technique	72402	Spinal stenosis, lumbar region, without neurogenic claudication	Lower Back (Lumbar)	8	9,606	720,676	217,241

Table 4b. Average Costs and Number of People by CPTs, ICD-9 Codes, Body Regions– Outpatient Services

Procedure Codes		ICD-9	Diagnosis	Body Regions	N	Minimum Cost	Maximum Cost	Average Cost
C1820	Generator, neurostimulator (implantable), with rechargeable battery and charging system	72283	Postlaminectomy syndrome of lumbar region	Lower Back (Lumbar)	31	0	80596.06	26425.43
C1820	Generator, neurostimulator (implantable), with rechargeable battery and charging system	72252	Degeneration of lumbar or lumbosacral intervertebral disc	Lower Back (Lumbar)	6	10178.25	55502.34	24883.55
L8687	Implantable neurostimulator pulse generator, dual array, rechargeable, includes extension	72283	Postlaminectomy syndrome of lumbar region	Lower Back (Lumbar)	12	0	43188	22069.18
J1745	Injection infliximab, 10 mg	72190	Spondylosis of unspecified site with myelopathy	Nonspecific	8	2582.129	112565.3	20668
L8699	Prosthetic implant, not otherwise specified	73730	Scoliosis (and kyphoscoliosis) idiopathic	Nonspecific	6	0	40500	17925.09
L8699	Prosthetic implant, not otherwise specified	72402	Spinal stenosis, lumbar region, without neurogenic claudication	Lower Back (Lumbar)	17	3.83	57563.34	17057.81
C1772	Infusion pump, programmable (implantable)	72283	Postlaminectomy syndrome of lumbar region	Lower Back (Lumbar)	9	0	37656.88	16020.6

Table 4b. (Continued)

Procedure Codes		ICD-9	Diagnosis	Body Regions	N	Minimum Cost	Maximum Cost	Average Cost
63056	Transpedicular approach with decompression of spinal cord, equina and/or nerve root(s) (e.g., herniated intervertebral disc), single segment; lumbar (including transfacet, or lateral extraforaminal approach) (e.g., far lateral herniated intervertebral disc)	72273	Intervertebral disc disorder with myelopathy lumbar region	Lower Back (Lumbar)	27	201.0099	55000	14999.4
63030	lumbar discectomy [laminotomy (hemilaminectomy), with decompression of nerve root(s), including partial facetectomy, foraminotomy and/or excision of herniated intervertebral disc, 1 interspace, lumbar]	72283	Postlaminectomy syndrome of lumbar region	Lower Back (Lumbar)	10	216.36	84168.88	14082.27
L8699	Prosthetic implant, not otherwise specified	72252	Degeneration of lumbar or lumbosacral intervertebral disc	Lower Back (Lumbar)	10	6.389999	29087.45	13823.16

Legend: Tables 4a and 4b. Average Costs by DRG, procedure, and ICD-9 codes. The top ten DRG codes with the highest average costs per person are presented with inpatient data in Table 4a and the top ten procedure codes with the highest average costs per person in the outpatient data are presented in Table 4b. Average costs per person were assessed in the inpatient data by DRG code, then results with only one observation were removed, and the results ordered by average cost. Similarly, outpatient data was analyzed for average costs per person by procedure code, results with only one observation excluded, and remaining results ordered by average cost. Procedure codes and ICD-9 codes associated with the DRG code are listed in Table 4a, and the ICD-9 code associated with the procedure code are listed in Table 4b.

In the fifty codes (20 of these are represented in Table 3b and the rest are in Appendix B) with the highest average costs per person, 12 codes were related to intervertebral disc disorders (N=1,190,877 individuals), 8 codes were for diagnoses related to the curvature of the spine (N=177,817), 2 codes were diagnoses for lumbar (predominantly) and thoracic stenosis (N=169,193), 11 codes were related to cervical and thoracic dislocation (N=131,396), 7 codes were related to postlaminectomy diagnoses (N=93,311), and 3 codes were related to spondylosis diagnoses (N=39,201). The diagnosis of other, pain disorder related to psychological factors occurred for 6,471 individuals with an outpatient average cost per person of $237,whereas those related to inpatient admissions was $36,411.

Tables 4a and 4b present analyses of average costs per person for DRG and procedure codes. These costs were calculated for the data analyzed in Tables 2 and 3 by DRG code, then costs in which only one observation was used to calculate the value were excluded, and then the data ordered by cost. Among the inpatient data, the analysis results of which are presented in Table 4a, the highest average cost per person by DRG code was for DRG code 454, combined anterior/posterior spinal fusion with complications and comorbidities, for 6 individuals in the dataset. This DRG code was associated with an MSD ICD-9 code of 737.30, scoliosis (and kyphoscoliosis) idiopathic. Among the top ten highest average cost per person DRG codes, nine were spinal fusion procedures associated with ICD-9 codes related to spinal curvature diagnoses. For the outpatient data, the average cost per person for the highest costing procedure code was for implantation of a generator, neurostimulators (implantable), with rechargeable battery and charging system, procedure code C1820, for 31 individuals in the dataset and association with an ICD-9 code of 722.83, postlaminectomy syndrome of lumbar region. Of the top ten highest average costs per person by procedure codes, presented in Table 4b, seven were for implantable neurostimulators or other devices, and two were for laminectomy procedures.

Multinomial logistic regression analysis evaluated differences across body region groups, incorporating the independent variables of gender, age groups, geographic location, industry type, and logarithm of total cost per person into models, using data for referenced ICD-9 codes. In these analyses, the referent group is female, age 35-44, works in the manufacturing/non-durable goods sector, and resides in the southern region of the US. These analyses, presented in Tables 5 (inpatient) and 6 (outpatient) indicate several differences across body region groups.

Table 5. Multinomial Logit Regression of Body Regions of Neck (Cervical), Upper Back (Thoracic), and Lower Back (Lumbar) Adjusting for Age, Gender, Geographic, and Industry Variables – Inpatient Analysis

Effect	Odds Ratio Point Estimate	95% Wald Confidence Limits	
Neck Body Region			
Male	1.95*	1.71	2.22
Oil, Gas and Mining	1.86*	1.17	2.
Manufacturing, Durable	1.15	.970	1.38
Transportation, Communication and Utilities	.884	.73	1.07
Retail	.957	.673	1.3
Finance, Insurance and Real estate	1.41*	1.15	1.73
North East	.796*	.645	.9
North Central	.620*	.523	.73
West	.718*	.612	.84
0 – 17 years	.031*	.021	.04
18 - 34 years	.184*	.144	.24
45 - 54 years	1.18	.989	1.42
55 - 64 years	.626*	.520	.75
Log(Total Cost)	.877*	.829	.93
Upper Back Body Region			
Male	1.88*	1.56	2.26
Oil, Gas and Mining	.81	.358	1.87
Manufacturing, Durable	1.10	.859	1.42
Transportation, Communication and Utilities	.98	.755	1.2
Retail	.519*	.272	.98
Finance, Insurance and Real estate	1.0	.741	1.37
North East	.917	.674	1.24
North Central	1.01	.801	1.28

Effect	Odds Ratio	95% Wald	
	Point Estimate	Confidence Limits	
West	.827	.652	1.04
0 – 17 years	.067*	.040	.11
18 - 34 years	.520*	.379	.71
45 - 54 years	1.21	.931	1.59
55 - 64 years	.814	.61	1.07
Log(Total Cost)	.936	.863	1.01
Lower Back Body Region			
Male	2.12*	1.92	2.34
Oil, Gas and Mining	1.24	.844	1.82
Manufacturing, Durable	1.2*	1.05	1.38
Transportation, Communication and Utilities	.937	.81	1.07
Retail	.949	.733	1.22
Finance, Insurance and Real estate	1.20*	1.03	1.41
North East	.904	.772	1.05
North Central	.918	.812	1.03
West	.794*	.705	.89
0 – 17 years	.013*	.010	.02
18 - 34 years	.310*	.265	.36
45 - 54 years	.981	.848	1.13
55 - 64 years	.736*	.638	.85
Log(Total Cost)	.718*	.688	.75

Legend. Table 5. Multinomial Logit Regression of Body Regions of Neck (Cervical), Upper Back (Thoracic), and Lower Back (Lumbar) Adjusting for Age, Gender, Geographic, and Industry Variables – Inpatient Analysis: The table presents the Relative Risk Ratios and confidence interval estimates for the inpatient data evaluated from the Medstat database, as described in the methods. Body regions are described in the methods. The referent group is female, age 35-44, works in the manufacturing/non-durable goods sector, and resides in the southern region of the US. The asterisks (*) signify the statistically significant outputs.

In the inpatient data (Table 5), increased relative risk ratios were found for males in all three body regions examined [neck: RRR = 1.95 (95% CI = 1.71, 2.22); upper back: RRR = 1.88 (95% CI = 1.56, 2.26); and lower back: RRR = 2.12 (95% CI = 1.92, 2.34)].

Geographic location in the north or west is associated with fewer neck related diagnoses, and location in the west was protective compared to the referent group for lower back diagnoses. Age less than 34 or age 55-64 was associated with fewer neck and lower back diagnoses, as was age less than 34 with upper back.

Finance, insurance, and real estate workers had significantly more neck and lower back diagnoses than workers in the manufacturing of durable goods who had lower rates of back diagnoses. Retail workers had fewer thoracic diagnoses compared to the referent group consisting of female, age 35 – 44 years. The logarithm of cost variable indicated that the referent group was less likely to have higher costs than males in the inpatient admissions data with respect to neck and lower back diagnoses.

In the outpatient data (Table 6), increased relative risk ratios were found for males in all three body regions examined [neck: relative risk ratio (RRR) = 1.27 (95% Confidence Interval (CI) = 1.25, 1.28); upper back: RRR = 1.57 (95% CI = 1.55, 1.59); and lower back: RRR = 1.85 (95% CI = 1.83, 1.87)]. Geographic locations in the north or west were associated with more neck and upper back related diagnoses.

Age less than 34 or greater than 45 was associated with fewer neck and upper back diagnoses. In the lower back, increased RRRs were found for all industries except for transportation/communication/utilities and finance/insurance/real estate workers.

In the lower back, more lumbar diagnoses were associated with northcentral geographic location and age between 45 and 54, while age below 34 was associated with fewer lumbar diagnoses, and age 55-64 was not significantly different from the referent group. The logarithm of cost variable indicated that the referent group was less likely to have higher costs than males in the outpatient services data.

Table 6. Multinomial Logit Regression of Body Regions of Neck (Cervical), Upper Back (Thoracic), and Lower Back (Lumbar) Adjusting for Age, Gender, Geographic, and Industry Variables – Outpatient Analysis

Effect	Odds Ratio	95% Wald	
	Point Estimate	Confidence Limits	
Neck Body Region			
Male	1.27*	1.25	1.28
Oil, Gas and Mining	.67*	.63	.71
Manufacturing, Durable	.76*	.75	.77
Transportation, Communication and Utilities	.634*	.62	.64
Retail	.625*	.59	.65
Finance, Insurance and Real estate	.601*	.58	.61
North East	1.38*	1.34	1.4
North Central	6.10*	6.0	6.20
West	1.25*	1.23	1.28
0 – 17 years	.8*	.08	.08
18 - 34 years	.55*	.54	.56
45 - 54 years	.94*	.92	.96
55 - 64 years	.66*	.65	.68
Log(Total Cost)	1.07*	1.07	1.08
Upper Back Body Region			
Male	1.57*	1.55	1.59
Oil, Gas and Mining	.90*	.85	.96
Manufacturing, Durable	.700*	.69	.72
Transportation, Communication and Utilities	.92*	.90	.94
Retail	.68*	.65	.72
Finance, Insurance and Real estate	.66*	.65	.68
North East	1.08*	1.06	1.11

Table 6. (Continued)

Effect	Odds Ratio	95% Wald	
	Point Estimate	Confidence Limits	
North Central	3.09*	3.03	3.14
West	1.44*	1.42	1.47
0 – 17 years	.08*	.08	.08
18 - 34 years	.67*	.65	.68
45 - 54 years	.92*	.89	.94
55 - 64 years	.72*	.71	.74
Log(Total Cost)	1.07*	1.07	1.08
Lower Back Body Region			
Male	1.85*	1.83	1.87
Oil, Gas and Mining	1.14*	1.10	1.1
Manufacturing, Durable	1.04*	1.03	1.05
Transportation, Communication and Utilities	1.0*	1.00	1.03
Retail	1.07*	1.05	1.11
Finance, Insurance and Real estate	.94*	.93	.958
North East	.935*	.92	.95
North Central	1.56*	1.54	1.58
West	.80*	.79	.81
0 – 17 years	.02*	.02	.02
18 - 34 years	.45*	.45	.46
45 - 54 years	1.08*	1.06	1.10
55 - 64 years	1.01*	.99	1.03
Log(Total Cost)	1.07*	1.07	1.08

Legend. Table 6: Multinomial Logit Regression of Body Regions of Neck (Cervical), Upper Back (Thoracic), and Lower Back (Lumbar) Adjusting for Age, Gender, Geographic, and Industry Variables – Outpatient Analysis: The table presents the Relative Risk Ratios and confidence interval estimates for the outpatient data evaluated from the Medstat database, as described in the methods. Body regions are described in the methods. The referent group is female, age 35-44, works in the manufacturing/non-durable goods sector, and resides in the southern region of the US. The asterisks (*) signify the statistically significant outputs.

Discussion

Average costs per person among the three body regions of focus in this analysis were found to be highest for upper back in the inpatient data and for lower back in the outpatient data. Approximately half (25 out of 47) ICD-9 codes with the highest average costs per person in the inpatient data consisted of intervertebral disc, spinal stenosis, and scoliosis codes. Of the outpatient service records examined, 23 out of 50 codes were for intervertebral disc, spinal curvature, and spinal stenosis diagnoses. The highest average costs among the DRG codes were those related to spinal fusion, and among procedural codes those related to implantable devices (e.g. generators and neurostimulators). Regression analysis across body regions, accounting for demographic, work, and total cost variables, revealed several key findings. Evaluation based on extraction of records of inpatient and outpatient data suggests that males have greater risk ratios for diagnoses in all three body regions examined. This might be due, for example, to greater exposure of males to hazardous environments, in comparison to females, causing higher MSD, although the current analysis does not allow definitive determination of cause. Geographic location had a range of effects on risk for cervical, thoracic, and lumbar diagnoses. There were fewer significant effects of industry type in the inpatient data. The effects of industry reflects decreased risk ratios relative to the manufacturing non-durable goods sector in the outpatient data. Average costs were greater for the referent group in the inpatient data for neck and lower back, but were decreased for the referent group in the outpatient data across all three body regions.

The outcomes obtained differ between the inpatient and outpatient claims. The outpatient claims analysis signifies that employees residing in the north central part are more likely to have MSD. MSD in lower back regions are more prevalent among those employed in the retail trade sector. The inpatient medical claims analysis suggests that male individuals are more likely to have MSD, and that those employed in the oil, gas and mining industry are more likely to have neck and lower back related medical claims and those in the age group of 45 to 54 years are more likely to have neck and upper back related MSD. The analysis of medical costs in administrative databases related to MSD classified by ICD-9, DRG and procedure codes are less well-developed in the literature. This study contributes to the literature of medical costs of MSD focusing on different medical cost components as well as demographic factors. The use of a medical claims dataset has certain advantages and challenges. Conclusions drawn from analysis of this data potentially have more generalizability due to the broader demographic characteristics of the data set, particularly with respect to geographic location and age. Examination of employed individuals may increase the relevance of the findings for working populations. Such data sets, however, also are subject to significant oversight and management to ensure integrity of the data (Thompson Reuters, 2010). Claims data, however, present challenges with respect to ascertainment of diagnostic and procedural codes used for data selection and analysis (Clement et al, 2013; Benchimol et al., 2011). In particular, the use of ICD-9 and other diagnostic and procedural codes to select cases for analysis of health impacts and costs requires, ideally, the use of validated codes. The availability of validated codes would potentially mitigate the risk for selection bias that could influence results. Validation could be by methods such as multiple researchers independently selecting codes to best choose cases, with a consensus built from such exercises and adequate statistical analysis of reproducibility (Walraven et al., 2012) or the use of published codes combined from previous studies that may have a published literature supporting the accuracy of such codes to correctly select cases, a "referenced" set of identifying codes (Sinnot et al., 2012).

Future considerations include methodologic and hypothesis related developments including a broader range of outcomes, wage replacement payments, days away from work and a broader range of MSD conditions. Differences due to identification of records by ICD-9 codes or other codes as well as differences in health care access/utilization, versus differences due to prevalence/incidence of different diagnoses, are both potential explanations for findings in studies of health effects and costs in administrative databases. Improved methods of selecting cases, for example, that include ICD-9, DRG and procedural codes, as well as other markers of diagnosis, may address some of this issue. Using validated or referenced versus non-validated or non-referenced codes to examine datasets and extract records for analyses may also be important to understand variables related to MSD and associated costs. Use of a variable such as body region, as utilized in this analysis, requires further evaluation as a method of classifying data to compare factors associated with MSD and costs. The role of variables such as industry type and geographic location also require further evaluation, along with standard demographic variables such as age and gender. Such methods development would contribute to improved analyses of MSD related health effects, industry and other characteristics, and costs in administrative databases, and allow for more refined evaluation of issues specific to employed individuals with MSD.

Appendix – A
Average Costs by ICD-9 Codes, Body Regions–Inpatient Admissions

ICD-9	Diagnosis	Body Region	N	Minimum Cost	Maximum Cost	Average Cost
73712	Kyphosis postlaminectomy	Nonspecific	7	45,416	216,767	92,222
72401	Spinal stenosis of thoracic region	Upper Back (Thoracic)	78	360	572,162	88,498
72251	Degeneration of thoracic or thoracolumbar intervertebral disce	Upper Back (Thoracic)	137	926	1,264,538	86,124
72141	Spondylosis with myelopathy thoracic region	Upper Back (Thoracic)	35	2,885	357,910	85,029
72270	Intervertebral disc disorder with myelopathy unspecified region	Nonspecific	13	9,608	566,675	73,061
72292	Other and unspecified disc disorder of thoracic region	Upper Back (Thoracic)	53	2,786	398,153	70,347
72402	Spinal stenosis, lumbar region, without neurogenic claudication	Lower Back (Lumbar)	4791	9	1,461,554	67,680
73742	Lordosis associated with other conditions	Lower Back (Lumbar)	6	10,231	150,661	63,898
72283	Postlaminectomy syndrome of lumbar region	Lower Back (Lumbar)	422	1,032	660,350	63,154
72252	Degeneration of lumbar or lumbosacral intervertebral disc	Lower Back (Lumbar)	3183	-	937,716	59,709
72293	Other unspecified disc disorder of lumbar region	Lower Back (Lumbar)	597	300	712,957	58,713
72271	Intervertebral disc disorder with myelopathy cervical region	Neck (Cervical)	1192	1,116	932,630	58,708
72273	Intervertebral disc disorder with myelopathy lumbar region	Lower Back (Lumbar)	372	43	709,015	58,518

Appendix A. (Continued)

ICD-9	Diagnosis	Body Region	N	Minimum Cost	Maximum Cost	Average Cost
72211	Displacement of thoracic intervertebral disc without myelopathy	Upper Back (Thoracic)	160	175	800,480	56,299
72142	Spondylosis with myelopathy lumbar region	Lower Back (Lumbar)	48	2,708	207,947	54,159
72281	Postlaminectomy syndrome of cervical region	Neck (Cervical)	67	2,847	302,876	53,636
72291	Other and unspecified disc disorder of cervical region	Neck (Cervical)	507	801	1,491,176	53,380
72290	Other and unspecified disc disorder of unspecified region	Nonspecific	117	514	406,428	52,702
72280	Postlaminectomy syndrome of unspecified region	Nonspecific	25	1,315	368,321	52,026
83920	Closed dislocation lumbar vertebra	Lower Back (Lumbar)	44	5,725	313,470	48,046
72190	Spondylosis of unspecified site without myelopathy	Nonspecific	176	744	353,982	43,062
30789	Other, pain disorder related to psychological factors	Nonspecific	102	1,478	379,920	36,411
72210	Displacement of lumbar intervertebral disc without myelopathy	Lower Back (Lumbar)	3356	-	843,837	32,850
73720	Lordosis (acquired) (postural)	Nonspecific	39	4,292	292,245	32,497
72479	Other disorders of coccyx	Lower Back (Lumbar)	53	774	222,827	29,348
72232	Schmorl's nodes of lumbar region	Upper Back (Thoracic)	7	2,173	66,102	24,754
72231	Schmorl's nodes of thoracic region	Neck (Cervical)	6	6,655	29,877	17,091

Appendix – B
Average Costs by ICD-9 Codes, Body Regions–Outpatient Services

ICD-9	Diagnosis	Body Region	N	Minimum Cost	Maximum Cost	Average Cost
72252	Degeneration of lumbar or lumbosacral intervertebral disc	Lower Back (Lumbar)	492565	0	290361	341.421
72281	Postlaminectomy syndrome of cervical region	Neck (Cervical)	15181	0	100555	337.6902
73719	Other kyphosis acquired	Nonspecific	717	0	17572.65	329.6016
72273	Intervertebral disc disorder with myelopathy lumbar region	Lower Back (Lumbar)	37048	0	72777.89	319.6333
72251	Degeneration of thoracic or thoracolumbar intervertebral disc	Upper Back (Thoracic)	27616	0	71394.88	306.6784
73739	Other kyphosis and scoliosis	Nonspecific	11152	0	162632	300.2871
73720	Lordosis (acquired) (postural)	Nonspecific	4104	0	34316.58	299.6638
73729	Other lordosis acquired	Nonspecific	678	0	7910	293.3985
83931	Open dislocation thoracic vertebra	Lower Back (Lumbar)	60	0	3071.729	289.9596
83912	Open dislocation second cervical vertebra	Neck (Cervical)	27	5.309998	4020.838	281.6054
72142	Spondylosis with myelopathy lumbar region	Lower Back (Lumbar)	9744	0	77088.5	280.4011
73710	Kyphosis (acquired) (postural)	Nonspecific	18260	0	72799.98	268.5505
72290	Other and unspecified disc disorder of unspecified region	Nonspecific	7744	0	59491.5	244.0819
72230	Schmorl's nodes of unspecified region	Nonspecific	308	0	2816.578	242.9027
30789	Other, pain disorder related to psychological factors	Nonspecific	6471	0	12997.27	237.9031

Appendix B. (Continued)

ICD-9	Diagnosis	Body Region	N	Minimum Cost	Maximum Cost	Average Cost
72270	Intervertebral disc disorder with myelopathy unspecified region	Nonspecific	1498	0	18592.73	235.9477
73730	Scoliosis (and kyphyscoliosis) idiopathic	Nonspecific	149902	0	217747.8	234.9686
73743	Scoliosis associated with other conditions	Nonspecific	7691	0	172250.1	221.6174
83930	Open dislocation lumbar vertebra	Upper Back (Thoracic)	251	0	3967.958	217.7314
73734	Thoracogenic scoliosis	Upper Back (Thoracic)	2889	0	19934.72	215.9835
83904	Closed dislocation of fourth cervical vertebra	Neck (Cervical)	3788	0	23953.47	214.7471
72190	Spondylosis of unspecified site without myelopathy	Nonspecific	27533	0	112565.3	213.4298
83921	Closed dislocation thoracic vertebra	Upper Back (Thoracic)	67470	0	45632.25	212.4443
83902	Closed dislocation second cervical vertebra	Neck (Cervical)	11014	0	36338.25	208.0394
83907	Closed dislocation seventh cervical vertebra	Neck (Cervical)	4870	0	114899.1	204.4013
83903	Closed dislocation third cervical vertebra	Neck (Cervical)	2379	0	10254	203.0481
83906	Closed dislocation sixth cervical vertebra	Neck (Cervical)	8089	0	47037.45	201.7781
73740	Unspecified curvature of spine associated with other conditions	Nonspecific	684	0	12500	200.1613
83905	Closed dislocation fifth cervical vertebra	Neck (Cervical)	15306	0	6400	196.6267
83901	Closed dislocation of first cervical vertebra	Neck (Cervical)	18353	0	5500	195.8997

Legend: Appendix A and B. Average Costs by ICD-9 Codes, Body Regions. The next 30 ICD-9 codes (21 - 50) with the highest average costs per person following Tables 3a and 3b are presented with inpatient data in Appendix A and outpatient data in Appendix B.

References

American Academy of Orthopedic Surgeons, 2008. United States Bone and Joint Decade: The Burden of Musculoskeletal Diseases in the United States.Rosemont IL .

American Academy of Orthopedic Surgeons. Burden of Musculoskeletal Disease project. Chapter 1 - Burden of Musculoskeletal Diseases Overview. Accessed online at http://www.boneandjointburden.org/pdfs/BMUS_chpt1_overview.pdf; August 5, 2014.

American Federation of Labor and Congress of Industrial Organizations (AFL-CIO)., 2012. Report on 'Death on the job, the toll of neglect: A national and state-by-state profile of worker safety and health in the United States'.

Andersson GBJ. Epidemiology of low back pain. *Acta Orthop Scand.* 1998;69 Suppl 281:28–31.

Baldwin M. Reducing the cost of workrelated musculoskeletal disorders: targeting 386 H. PIEDRAHITA JOSE 2006, Vol. 12, No. 4 strategies to chronic disability cases. *J Electromyogr Kinesiol.* 2004;14:33–41.

Beach TA, Parkinson RJ, Stothart JP, Callaghan JP. Effects of prolonged sitting on the passive flexion stiffness of the in vivo lumbar spine. *Spine J.* 2005 Mar-Apr;5(2):145-54.

Benchimol EI, Manuel DG, To T, Griffiths AM, Rabeneck L, Guttmann A. Development and use of reporting guidelines for assessing the quality of validation studies of health administrative data. *J Clin Epid.* 2011; 64:821-829.

Bhattacharya, Anasua "Costs of Occupational Musculoskeletal Disorders (MSD) in the United States", *International Journal of Industrial ergonomics,* 2014, 44(3): 448-454.

Bhattacharya, Anasua and J. Paul Leigh. "Musculoskeletal Disorder Costs and Medical Claim Filing in the US Retail Trade Sector." *Industrial Health,* 2011, 49: 517-22.

Blair S, Djupsjöbacka M, Johansson H, Ljubisavljevic M, Passatore M, Windhorst U, et al., Neuromuscular mechanisms behind chronic work-related myalgias: an overview. In: Johansson H, Windhorse U, Djupjöbacka M, Passatore M, editors. *Chronic work-related myalgia.* Neuromuscular mechanisms behind work-related chronic muscle syndromes. Gävle, Sweden: Gävle University Press; 2003. p. 5–46.

Brogmus, G.E., Sorock, G.S., Webster, B.S., 1996. Recent Trends in Work-Related Cumulative Trauma Disorders of the Upper Extremities in the United States: An Evaluation of Possible Reasons. *Journal of Occupational and Environmental Medicine* 38(4), 401-11.

Brooks PM. The burden of musculoskeletal disease – a global perpective. *Clin Rheumato*l. 2006; 25:778-781.

Bureau of Labor Statistics (BLS), 2011. Nonfatal Occupational Injuries and Illnesses Requiring Days Away from Work, 2010. Available from: http://www.bls.gov/news.release/osh2.nr0.htm (Accessed Sept 10, 2014).

Bureau of Labor Statistics (BLS). 2012, Lost-worktime injuries and illnesses: characteristics and resulting time away from work (2012). Washington, DC, USA: U.S. Department of Labor; 2013.

Bureau of Labor Statistics (BLS). Nonfatal occupational injuries and illnesses requiring days away from work, 2012. USDL-13-2257; November 26, 2013. Accessed online at http://www.bls.gov/news.release/pdf/osh2.pdf http://www.bls.gov/news.release/pdf/osh2.pdf Accessed on Aug. 15, 2014.

Clement ND, Murray IR, Nie YX, McBirnie JM. Cracking the code: the accuracy of coding shoulder procedures and the repercussions. Scottish Medical Journal. 2013; 58 (2): 109-112.

De Coster C, Quan H, Finlayson A, Gao M, Halfon P, Humphries KH, Johansen H, Lix, LM, Luthi JC, Roman PS, Roos L, Sundararajan V, Tu JV, Webster G, Chali WA. Identifying priorities in methodlogical research using ICD-9-CM and ICD-10 administrative data: report form an international consortium. *BMC Health Services Research.* 2006; 6:77-82.

Driscoll T. Epidemiological aspects of studying work-related musculoskeletal disorders. *Best Practice & Res Clin Rheum.* 2011; 25:3-13.

Dunning, K.K., Davis, K.G., Cook, C., Kotowski, S.E., Hamrick, C., Jewell, G., Lockey, J., 2010. Costs by industry and diagnosis among musculoskeletal claims in a state workers compensation system: 1999-2004. *Am. J. Ind. Med.* 53(3), 276-84.

Ensor KL, Kwon YW, Dibeneditto MR, Zuckerman JD, Rokito AS. The rising incidence of rotator cuff repairs. *J Shoulder Elbow Surg.* 2013 Dec;22(12):1628-32. doi: 10.1016/j.jse.2013.01.006. Epub 2013 Mar 1

Freburger JK, Holmes GM, Agans RP, et al., The rising prevalence of chronic low back pain. Arch Intern Med. 2009;169(3):251-258.

Gardner, B.T., Dale, A.M., VanDillen, L., Franzblau, A. and Evanoff, B.A. (2008) Predictors of upper extremity symptoms and functional impairment among workers employed for 6 months in a new job. *American Journal of Industrial Medicine,* 51, 932-940.

Gore, Mugdha PhD, BPharm*; Sadosky, Alesia PhD†; Stacey, Brett R. MD‡; Tai, Kei-Sing MS*; Leslie, Douglas PhD§ The Burden of Chronic Low Back Pain: Clinical Comorbidities, Treatment Patterns, and Health Care Costs in Usual Care Settings, Spine: 15 May 2012 - Volume 37 - Issue 11 - p E668–E677 doi: 10.1097/BRS.0b013e318241e5de.0 *Health Services Research*

Guo HR, Takana S, Halperin WE, Cameron LL. Back pain prevalence in US industry and estimates of lost workdays. Am J Public Health. 1999;89(7):1029–35.

Hashemi, L., Webster, B.S., Clancy, E.A., Courtney, T.K., 1998. Length of Disability and Cost of Work-Related Musculoskeletal Disorders of the Upper Extremity. *J. Occup. Environ. Med.* 40, 261-9.

Katz JN. Lumbar disc disorders and low-back pain: socioeconomic factors and consequences [review]. *J Bone Joint Surg Am.* 2006;88(suppl 2):21-24.

Kostanjsek N, Escorpizo R, Boonen A, Walsh NE, Ustün TB, Stucki G. Assessing the impact of musculoskeletal health conditions using the International Classification of Functioning, Disability and Health. Disabil Rehabil. 2011;33(13-14):1281-97. doi: 10.3109/09638288.2010.526165. *Epub* 2010 Oct 14

Leigh J, Macaskill P, Kuosma E, Mandryk J. Global burden of diseases and injuries due to occupational factors. *Epidemiology.* 1999;10(5):626–31.

Leigh, J.P., Markowitz, S.B., Fahs, M.C., Landrigan, P.J., 2000. Costs of Occupational Injuries and Illnesses. Ann Arbor: Univ. of Michigan Press.

Luttmann, A., Jäger, M., Griefahn, B., Caffier, G., Liebers, F. and Steinberg, U. (2003). *Preventing musculoskeletal disorders in the workplace: Protecting workers' health series No. 5.* World Health Organisation.

Morse, T., Dillon, C., Warren, N., Levestain, C., Warren A., 1998. The economic and social consequences of work-related musculoskeletal disorders: the Connecticut upper-extremity surveillance project (CUSP). *Int. J. Occup. Med. Environ. Health*, 4:209–16.

National Research Council and Institute of Medicine, 2001. Musculoskeletal disorder and workplace: low back and upper extremities. Panel on musculoskeletal disorder and the workplace. Washington, DC, USA: National Academic Press.

Osborne A, Blake C, Fullen BM, Meredith D, Phelan J, McNamara J, Cunningham C. Prevalence of musculoskeletal disorders among farmers: A systematic review. Am J Ind Med. 2012 Feb;55(2):143-58. doi: 10.1002/ajim.21033. *Epub* 2011 Nov 8.

Peele, P.B., Xu, Y., Colombi, A., 2005. Medical care and lost work day costs in musculoskeletal disorders: Older versus younger workers. *International Congress Series* 1280, 214–8.

Piedrahita, H., 2006. Costs of Work-Related Musculoskeletal Disorders (MSD) in Developing Countries: Colombia Case. *International Journal of Occupational Safety and Ergonomics (JOSE),* 12(4), 379–386.

Riihimäki H, Kurppa K, Karjalainen A, Palo L, Jolanki R, Keskinen H, et al., Occupational diseases in Finland in 2002: new cases of occupational diseases reported to the Finnish Register of Occupational Diseases. Helsinki, Finland: Finnish Institute of Occupational Health; 2004.

Rudolf KD, Kus S, Chung KC, Johnston M, LeBlanc M, Cieza A. Development of the International Classification of Functioning, Disability and Health core sets for hand conditions--results of the World Health Organization International Consensus process. Disabil Rehabil. 2012;34(8):681-93. doi: 10.3109/09638288.2011.613514. Epub 2011 Oct 6.

Saarni SI, Suvisaari J, Sintonen H, Koskinen S, Harkanen T, Lonnqvist J. The health-related quality-of-life impact of chronic conditions varied with age in general population. *J Clin Epid.* 2007; 60:1288-1297.

SAS Institute, Inc. Proprietary Software 9.3, licensed to US CENTERS FOR DISEASE CONTROL & PRVNTN. Copyright © 2002-2010 SAS Institute Inc. SAS and all other SAS Institute Inc. product or service names are registered trademarks or trademarks of SAS Institute Inc., Cary, NC, USA.

Sears JM, Blanar L, Bowman SM, Adams D, Silverstein BA. Predicting work-related disability and medical cost outcomes: estimating injury severity scores from workers' compensation data. *J Occup Rehabil.* 2013 Mar;23(1):19-31. doi: 10.1007/s10926-012-9377-x

Sengupta, I., Reno, V., Burton, J.F., 2009. Workers' Compensation: Benefits, Coverage, and Costs. Washington DC: National Academy of Social Insurance.

Silverstein, B., Adams, D., 2007. Work Related Musculoskeletal Disorders of the Neck, Back, and Upper Extremity in Washington State, 1997 – 2005. *Technical Report* Num. 40-11-2007, December 2007.

Sinnott PL, Siroka AM, Shane AC, Trafton JA, Wagner TH. Identifying neck and back pain in administrative data: defining the right cohort. Spine (Phila Pa 1976). 2012; May 1; 37(10):860-74. doi: 10.1097/ BRS.0b013e3182376508.

Sinnott PL, Wagner TH. Low back pain in VA users. *Arch Intern Med*, 2009; July 27; 169(14):1338-9.

StataCorp. 2013. *Stata Statistical Software: Release 13*. College Station, TX: StataCorp LP.

Straus BN. Chronic pain of spinal origin: the cost of intervention. Spine. 2002;27(22):2614–9.

Sveriges officiella statistik. Arnetsmiljö Verket. Occupational accidents and workrelated diseases (Statistik, rapport 2005:1. 2004). In Swedish with a summary in English. Retrieved October 9, 2006 from: http://www.xn--arbetsmiljverket-vwb.se/dokument/statistik/english/Occupational_2004.pdf.

Tanaka, S., Petersen, M.R., Cameron, L.L., 2001. Prevalence and risk factors of tendinitis and related disorders of the distal upper extremity among US workers: comparison to carpal tunnel syndrome, *American Journal of Industrial Medicine* 39, 328–335.

Timpka T, Jacobsson J, Bickenbach J, Finch CF, Ekberg J, Nordenfelt L. What is a sports injury? *Sports Med.* 2014 Apr;44(4):423-8. doi: 10.1007/s40279-014-0143-4.

Van Walvern C, Austen P. Administrative database research has unique characteristics that can risk biased results. *J of Clin Epid.* 2012; 65:126-131.

Van Walvern C, Bennet C, Forster AJ. Administrative database research infrequently used validated diagnostic or procedural codes. *J of Clin Epid.* 2011; 64:1054-1059.

Violante FS, Fiori M, Fiorentini C, Risi A, Garagnani G, Bonfiglioli R, Mattioli S. Associations of psychosocial and individual factors with three different categories of back disorder among nursing staff. *J Occup Health.* 2004 Mar;46(2):100-8.

Vos T, Flaxman AD, Naghavi M, et al., Years lived with disability (YLDs) for 1160 sequelae of 289 diseases and injuries 1990–2010: a systematic analysis for the Global Burden of Disease Study 2010. *Lancet* 2012;380:2163–96.

Webster, B.S., Snook S.H., 1994. The cost of compensable upper extremity cumulative trauma disorders. *J. Occup. Med.* 36,713-717. [Context Link]

Williams DA, Feuerstein M, Durbin D, Pezzullo J. Health care and indemnity costs across the natural history of disability in occupational low back pain. *Spine.* 1998;23(21):2329–36.

Woolf AD, Erwin J, March L. The need to address the burden of musculoskeletal conditions. *Best Practice & Res Clin Rheum*. 2012; 26:183-224.

Woolf AD, Vos T, March L. How to measure the impact of musculoskeletal conditions. *Best Practice & Res Clin Rheum*. 2010; 24:723-732.

Woolf, A.D., Pfleger, B., 2003. *Bulletin of the World Health Organization* 81(9), 646-56.

In: Musculoskeletal Diseases
Editor: Greg Reed

ISBN: 978-1-63463-551-6

Chapter II

Application of Differential Scanning Calorimetry for the Diagnosis of Musculoskeletal Diseases

N. Wiegand[1], L. G. Nöt[1], Z. Kiss[1] and D. Lőrinczy[2,*]

[1]Dept. of Traumatology and Hand Surgery, Faculty of Medicine, University of Pécs, Hungary

[2]Dept. of Biophysics, Faculty of Medicine, University of Pécs, Pécs, Hungary

Abstract

Background: Despite of the improved biochemical analyzes and imaging technology, diagnosis of different types of musculoskeletal diseases is still challenging. New methods are needed to improve the diagnostic procedures and help to select the most sufficient treatment.

Aims: The purpose of our current review was to demonstrate the usefulness of differential scanning calorimetry in the intraoperative diagnosis of musculoskeletal diseases.

* Corresponding author: Prof. Dr. Lőrinczy Dénes, Dept. of Biophysics, Faculty of Medicine, University of Pécs, H-7624, Pécs, Szigeti street 12. Hungary, e-mail: denes.lorinczy@aok.pte.hu.

Materials and methods: Different types of ligaments, connective tissues, joint capsules, arthritic or septic hyaline cartilage were collected intra operatively from pathologic, or healthy human origin. The thermal denaturation of the samples was monitored by a SETARAM Micro DSC-II calorimeter.

Results: Here we demonstrated a significant difference in the pattern of the thermal denaturation characteristics of the degenerative or inflamed collagen tissue samples, compared with the healthy human connective tissue. The degenerative samples' thermal enthalpy was significantly decreased, while the melting temperature showed an increase. In case of the inflamed samples, we found a significant increase in the enthalpy and a decrease of melting temperature.

Conclusion: These data suggest that DSC analysis could be a clinically relevant, additional method in the intraoperative diagnosis of different types of musculoskeletal diseases.

Keywords: Degenerative, inflammatory, cartilage, muscle, DSC (differential scanning calorimetry)

1. Introduction

The different types of musculoskeletal disorders affect millions of people worldwide. Despite of the recent advances in the pre-operative diagnostic procedures, to reach the correct diagnosis and establish the stage of certain degenerative and inflammatory diseases still could be challenging [1, 2]. Therefore, there is still a need for new methods to further support the accurate diagnosis of musculoskeletal diseases [1, 2]. Of the numerous cellular components of ligaments, joints and muscles, collagens were chosen as a primary target for our experiments. It is known that collagens are one of the elementary components of musculoskeletal system, ubiquitously found in all of the connective tissues. However, it is important to note, that of the 25 different types collagens, 90% of the collagen is type I, as an abundant component of skin, tendon, vascular ligature and bone. Additionally, type II collagen composes a dominant part of hyaline cartilage and collagen type III is found in granulation tissues [3-8]. Therefore, detection of level of structural changes of collagens due to degenerative or inflammatory diseases could be a useful diagnostic tool of several musculoskeletal disorders [1, 3-8]. The selection of musculoskeletal diseases included in our study was based on their high incidence and impact on the health condition of a relatively large proportion of population [1, 2, 6]. In the group of *degenerative diseases*, our primary selection involved ligaments, muscle tendons and hyaline cartilages [3, 7]. According to the literature, the connective tissue disorders of the hand have shown a significant increase in the last decades. Therefore, in the group *inflammatory* diseases, we focused to the carpal tunnel syndrome (CTS), De Quervain tenosynovitis and Dupuytren disease, with a common in pathomechanism: all of these syndromes are reported to be caused by a chronic, non-specific inflammation [8]. Here we also examined structural changes of the collagen, collected from muscle tissue, in diseases accompanied with cerebral palsy and congenital clubfoot in childhood [9]. The differential scanning calorimetry (DSC) measures the amount of heat required to increase the temperature over the time and compares with a standard reference sample. DSC is the only technique by which one can follow directly the change of heat capacity measured at constant pressure (C_P), which can monitor the actual state of the investigated structure. The acquired scans provide further data to determine the investigated tissue samples' enthalpy and melting temperature, described as the thermal characteristics. According to the thermal characteristics, the changes of enthalpy and melting temperature could be matched with the level structural damage of different proteins [10]. Despite of numerous *in vitro* or animal experiments, the DSC have been rarely used for analyzes of intra-operatively collected human tissue samples [11-13]. Meanwhile, in the past years, our workgroup has successfully utilized differential scanning calorimetry for the intra-operative diagnosis and staging of a wide variety of degenerative and inflammatory musculoskeletal diseases [4, 5, 8, 14-21]. Therefore, the goal of our current study is to provide evidence that comparison of thermal characteristics based on differential scanning calorimetry measurements could be a useful additional tool to achieve precise intra-operative diagnosis of different types of inflammatory and degenerative musculoskeletal disorders. Importantly, the accurate diagnosis and staging could be helpful in the choice of the most sufficient treatment.

2. Materials and Methods

2.1. Sample Preparation

In preparation and process of different samples, authors have attempted to follow a relatively standardized protocol [22]. However, different types of tissue samples and importantly, different circumstances of collection required the adjustment of our preparation and storage protocol. Despite of certain adjustments, it is need to be emphasized that those differences are not interfering with the comparative analyzes of the thermal characteristics of tissue samples with different origins.

Generally, the different types of healthy tissue samples were of mostly cadaver origin. The donors taken into our study were all under age of 45 at their death; considered to be free of any degenerative changes or chronic inflammatory diseases. These samples were only processed further in case degenerative or posttraumatic changes could not be verified macroscopically. The different types of pathologic tissue samples were all derived intra-operatively. Both control and pathologic samples were analyzed within the same time frames.

In case of *lower limb tendons,* the healthy human tendons were of cadaver origin and processed further only in case degeneration or post-traumatic changes of the tendons could not be verified macroscopically. The pathologic tendons were derived during surgical treatment of the Achilles, quadriceps tendon and patellar ligament ruptures. During the operations from we cut out roughly 1x2cm long samples from the already degenerated parts. Then, the ruptured ends of the tendons were connected surgically. The average age were 48 (32-61) years, relatively matching with the age of the cadavers.

For the *biceps tendon* measurements, all the samples were obtained during autopsy within 24 h post-mortem. We dissected the shoulder and the rotator cuff carefully, the rotator cuff lesions were evaluated, and the intra-articular portion of the LHB (long head of biceps) near to the bicipital groove was removed. The cadavers with macroscopic signs of rotator cuff pathology, or systemic metabolic disease such as diabetes as well as anamnesis of systemic corticosteroid medication were excluded from this study.

During the sample preparation of *degenerative femoral head and neck fractures*, we utilized a slightly different protocol for sample collection and storage. In this study, the healthy and pathologic human samples were derived from tissue fragments taken during operations and considered to be waste material. The donors of the control group taken into our study were all between the age of 65 and 75 females without symptoms of osteoarthritis. All of them suffered a Garden III or IV type femoral fractures and underwent a hip hemiprosthesis implantation within 12 hours after the accident. During the operations degenerative changes in their joints surface could not be verified macroscopically. The donors of the pathologic (avascular necrosis) group taken into the study were similar to the control group. They were all between the age of 65 and 75 females, they suffered a Garden III or IV femoral neck fractures too and they were free of osteoarthritis before the accident. Their fractures treated primary with cannulated screw fixation and during the post-operative period an avascular necrosis developed in their femoral head. The avascular necroses were proven with X-ray, CT or MR investigations. The second operations (hemiprosthesis) and sample preparations were performed within 1 and 20 months after the accident. The samples were obtained by devices especially designed for this task, from the same anatomic region (weight bearing surface of the femoral head) by standard methods both in the healthy and pathologic patient samples. The shape of samples was square with 5 mm of length and contained the full thickness of the cartilage without any bone tissue. Samples were washed three times in PBS (sterile phosphate-buffered saline, pH 7.4) in order to eliminate all of the remaining other tissue-parts. Samples were then put into sterile physiologic saline solution. All the individual samples were stored separately at 4°C, no longer than 6h. Then samples were subjected to calorimetric measurement. We measured 5 samples from control group and 11 pathologic cartilages.

In case of the *hand*, the healthy palmar fascias of the human hand were of cadaver origin. Both side aponeuroses were removed from two cadaver hands. The donors taken into the study were all under age of 45 at their death, we considered these persons to be free any degenerative changes in their joints. Samples were taken only from hands where any other kind of degeneration of the aponeurosis or post-traumatic changes of the hand could not be verified macroscopically. The pathologic ligaments were derived during operations of different seriousness of Dupuytren disease. During the operations, the degenerated parts of the aponeurosis were prepared and removed in full thickness and length.

All the medical interventions were made according to the ethical regulations and approved by the ethical committee of the University of Pécs.

2.2. DSC Measurements

Detailed description of our standardized DSC protocol are found elsewhere [22]. Briefly, the thermal denaturation was performed within 6 hours of sample collection, using a SETARAM Micro DSC-II calorimeter. All the experiments were performed between 0 and 100 °C. The heating rate was 0.3 K/min. Conventional Hastelloy batch vessels were used during the denaturation experiments with 850 μL sample volume (samples plus buffer) in average. Typical sample wet masses for calorimetric experiments were in between 100 – 200 mg. RPMI-1640 solution was used as a reference sample. We have plotted the C_P (DSC-II is a heat flux instrument with hermetically closed vessels) in the function of temperature. Calorimetric enthalpy was then calculated from the area under the $C_P(T)$ curve by using two-point setting SETARAM peak integration, and the data analyzed with OriginPro 7.5 after ASCII conversion.

2.3. Statistical Analysis

For statistical analyzes, unpaired two-way Student's t-test was used, with SPSS13.0 software (SPSS Inc., Chicago, IL). All data are expressed as mean. The statistically significant differences between groups were defined as $p < 0.05$.

3. Results

3.1. Comparison of the Thermal Characteristics of Degenerative and Intact Tissue Samples

In case of the degenerative tissue samples, we have found a significant increase of the thermal enthalpy, while the melting temperature showed mostly a moderate, but non-significant increase (Table I.). Based on our results, the Achilles tendon was found to be the less stable of all examined degenerative samples, with the higher level of decrease in the thermal enthalpy (ΔH_{cal} intact: 8 J/g vs. degenerative: 1.5 J/g) (Figure 1.). The quadriceps tendon showed a moderate decrease (ΔH_{cal} intact: 6.27 J/g vs. degenerative: 1.53 J/g). Meanwhile, the decrease of enthalpy was relatively similar in case of patellar ligament (ΔH_{cal} intact: 4.36 J/g vs. degenerative: 0.97 J/g) and knee cruciate ligament (ΔH_{cal} intact: 5.06 J/g vs. degenerative: 1.55 J/g). Notably, the samples from menisci (ΔH_{cal} intact: 4.9 J/g vs. degenerative: 3.6 J/g, $p<0.05$) and annulus fibrosus (ΔH_{cal} intact: 0.84 J/g vs. degenerative: 0.46 J/g, $p<0.05$) showed the lowest decrease in enthalpy.

The cartilage samples collected from avascular necrotic femoral head and arthritic femur condyle demonstrated a moderate, but significant increase

(ΔH_{cal} intact: 2.87 J/g vs. arthrotic: 4.02 J/g, $p<0.05$; ΔH_{cal} intact: 0.32 J/g vs. arthrotic: 0.58 J/g, $p<0.05$, respectively). In this set of experiments, cartilage samples were collected from patients who developed avascular necrosis of the femoral head (ANFH) after medial femoral neck fracture and screw fixation. At different time points following the primary surgery and depending on the onset of ANFH, the samples were taken intra-operatively during hip replacement. Interestingly, instead of the single thermal domain of the intact hyaline cartilage, we obtained on the DSC curves of the pathologic cartilages a wide endothermic transition (Figure 2.). In the cases of serious ANFH (6 months after the fracture), two different thermal domains appeared on the DSC scans. It could be the sign of severe damage of the cartilage, the denaturation of proteins and a formation of calcium deposits. However, arthritic patellar cartilage showed a significant decrease in both melting temperature and thermal enthalpy T_m intact: 64.8 J ^{0}C vs. arthritic: 6.90 ^{0}C, $p<0.05$; ΔH_{cal} intact: 1.78 J/g vs. arthritic: 0.78 J/g, $p<0.05$).

Table 1. The characteristic thermal parameters of the denaturation of different types of intact and degenerative human collagen structures

		Intact			Degenerative		
		n	T_m (^{0}C)	ΔH_{cal} (J/g)	n	T_m (^{0}C)	ΔH_{cal} (J/g)
1	Glenohumeral joint capsule	4	65.1	6.7	5	65.3	3.7*
2	Quadriceps tendon	4	63.3	6.27	5	64.8	1.53*
3	Patella tendon	4	61.7	4.36	4	63.9	0.97*
4	Achilles tendon	4	59.7	8.5	5	62.8	1.5*
5	Biceps tendon	12	63.4	6	16	62.9	1.28*
6	Knee cruciate ligament	4	64.8	5.06	5	65.1	1.55*
7	Meniscus	13	63.3	4.9	8	62.5	3.6*
8	Anulus fibrosus	14	60.5	0.84	18	62.5	0.46*
10	Femoral head avascular cartilage	5	68.2	2.87	9	70.8	4.02*
11	Femoral condyle arthrotic cartilage	3	72.6	0.32	6	58.9	0.58*
12	Patellar arthrotic cartilage	3	64.8	1.78	4	60.9	0.78*

n: number of samples, T_m (^{0}C): melting temperature, ΔH_{cal} (J/g): enthalpy. Unpaired Student's t-test, * indicates $p < 0.05$ vs. intact collagen samples. Data are expressed as mean, $n \geq 3$ in each group.

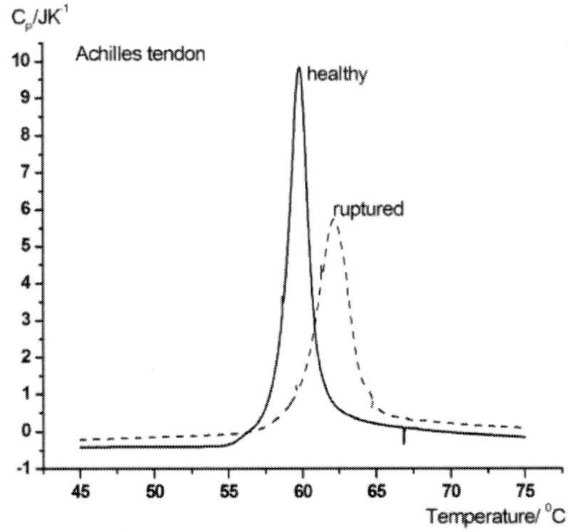

The endotherm processes are directed upward. The DSC curves represent significant alterations of the structure of ruptured Achilles tendon, indicated by the increased half width of denaturing temperature and decrease of calorimetric enthalpy.

Figure 1. Thermal denaturation scans of intact and ruptured human Achilles tendon.

3.2. Comparison of the Thermal Characteristics of Inflamed and Intact Tissue Samples

In contrast to the degenerative tissue samples, we have demonstrated a significant increase of the thermal enthalpy, comparing the inflamed and intact human tissue samples of patients with Dupuytren-contracture, De Quervain tenosynovitis and carpal tunnel syndrome (CTS) (Table 2.). The highest increase in the thermal enthalpy was found in case of carpal tunnel syndrome (ΔH_{cal} intact: 4.0 J/g vs. inflamed: 5.9 J/g, $p<0.05$) and De Quervian`s tenosynovitis (ΔH_{cal} intact: 3.84 J/g vs. inflamed: 5.39 J/g, $p<0.05$). Additionally, we found a less marked, but still significant increase in the enthalpy of samples from Dupuytren-contracture (ΔH_{cal} intact: 4.1 J/g vs. inflamed: 5.2 J/g). The acquired DSC scans clearly demonstrated significant changes between the different stages of the disease (Figure 3.). These changes were accompanied with a moderate, but not significant decrease in the denaturation temperature of samples collected from Dupuytren-contracture (Tm intact: 63.0 ^{0}C vs. inflamed: 61.7 ^{0}C) and also with a non-significant increase in samples from De Quervain tenosynovitis and carpal tunnel syndrome (T_m intact: 61.3 ^{0}C vs. degenerative: 62.1 ^{0}C; T_m intact: 61.3 ^{0}C vs. degenerative: 61.8 ^{0}C, respectively).

3.3. Comparison of the Thermal Characteristics of Injured and Intact Human Muscle Samples

Here we compared the standard calorimetric properties of the healthy human skeletal muscle with human skeletal muscles in primary peripheral leg deformities (congenital clubfeet) and secondary deformities caused by the malfunction of the central nervous system (cerebral palsy) (Table 3). The acquired data clearly demonstrate definitive changes in the enthalpy, comparing healthy controls to samples collected from patients with cerebral palsy or clubfoot deformity (ΔH_{cal} intact: 0.54 Jg^{-1}, cerebral palsy: 0.64 Jg^{-1}, clubfoot: 0.85 Jg^{-1}). It is important to note that healthy samples were collected during surgical correction of hallux valgus deformity; these samples were not from cadaver origin.

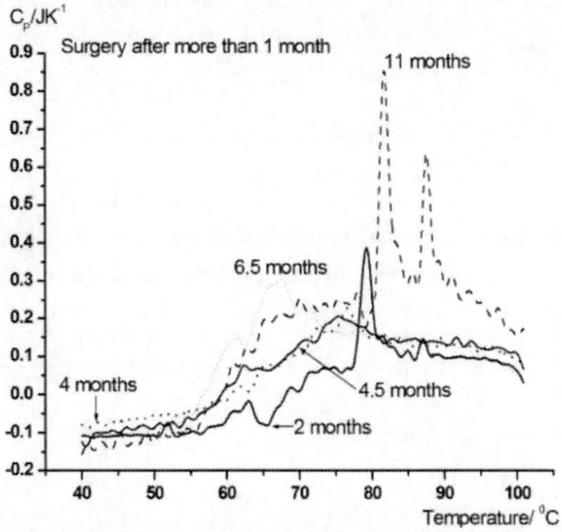

The endotherm processes are directed upward. The DSC scans clearly demonstrate significant differences between the samples collected at different time points after primary surgery. In cases of serious avascular necrosis (6 months after the fracture), two different thermal domains appear on the DSC scans.

Figure 2. Thermal denaturation scans of hyaline cartilage collected from patients with avascular necrosis of the femoral head (ANFH) at different time-points after primary surgery.

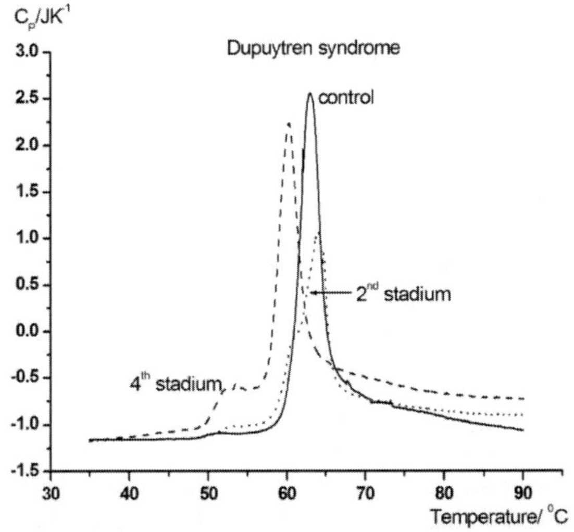

The endotherm processes are directed upward. The DSC scan indicate the presence of a single thermal domain with a weak water release after the denaturation. In Grade II, the presence of a second thermal structural unit can be observed that became more pronounced in Grade. IV. DSC scans clearly demonstrate the significant differences between the different stages, indicating the progression of the contracture.

Figure 3. Thermal denaturation scans of normal and clinically Grade II. and Grade IV. palmar fascia in Dupuytren disease.

Table 2. The characteristic thermal parameters of the denaturation of different types of intact and inflamed human collagen structures

		Intact			Inflamed		
		n	T_m (^{0}C)	ΔH_{cal} (J/g)	n	T_m (^{0}C)	ΔH_{cal} (J/g)
1	Dupuytren's contracture	4	63.0	4.1	10	61.7	5.2*
2	Carpal tunnel syndrome	4	61.3	4.0	10	61.8	5.9*
3	De Quervian`s tenosynovitis	4	61.3	3.84	10	62.1	5.39*

n: number of samples, T_m (^{0}C): melting temperature, ΔH_{cal} (J/g): enthalpy. Unpaired Student's t-test, * indicates $p < 0.05$ vs. intact collagen samples. Data are expressed as mean, $n \geq 3$ in each group.

Table 3. The characteristic thermal parameters of the denaturation of different types of intact and pathologic human muscle collagen structures

		Thermal parameters		
		n	T_m (^{0}C)	ΔH_{cal} (J/g)
1	Healthy control (adductor hallucis muscle)	3	56.5	0.54
2	Cerebral palsy (gastrocnemius muscle)	4	60.5	0.64
3	Clubfoot (adductor hallucis muscle)	4	57.7	0.85

n: number of samples, T_m (^{0}C): melting temperature, ΔH_{cal} (J/g): calorimetric enthalpy. Unpaired Student's t-test, * indicates $p < 0.05$ vs. healthy control collagen samples. Data are expressed as mean, $n \geq 3$ in each group.

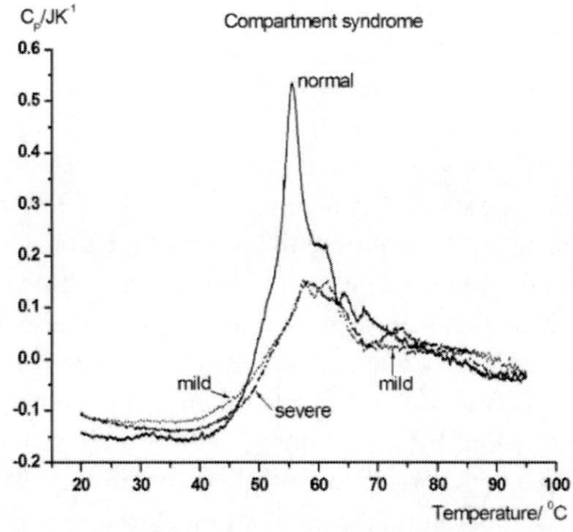

The endotherm processes are directed upward. The DSC scans showed no difference in the changes of heat capacity of native (healthy) and the denatured states of proteins depending on the stage of diseases. In case of control, we obtained a wide endothermic transition with two different thermal domains with T_ms 58.1 and 62.2 °C, that could be the melting of myosin and actin. In group I (mild stage), a significant change of the shape and melting temperatures (T_ms 55.5 and 59.9 °C) of denaturation were observed. The separation of myosin and actin contributions is more pronounced with a greater myosin enthalpy contribution, compared to the controls (indicated by the smaller half with of its thermal transition). In group II (severe stage), further transition temperature change can be observed (T_ms 57.45 and 61.5 °C) with increased myosin damage (smaller ΔH_{cal}), as a consequence of marked necrosis of the muscle.

Figure 4. Thermal denaturation scans of muscle samples from normal, mild and severe clinical stages of compartment syndrome.

With special clinical relevance, we also evaluated the changes of thermal characteristics of muscle samples, caused by compartment syndrome induced tissue ischemia. In case of the compartment syndrome, the DSC analyzes have demonstrated significant differences between the different types and severity grades of the collected samples (control: T_m: 55.5; 59.9 ^{0}C, ΔH_{cal}: 0.52 J/g, Gr. I.: T_m: 58.1; 62.2 ^{0}C, ΔH_{cal}: 0.28 J/g, Gr. II.: T_m: 57.45; 61.5 ^{0}C, ΔH_{cal}: 0.24 J/g, Volkmann's ischemic contracture: T_m: 57.75; 61.8; 65.8 ^{0}C and ΔH_{cal}: 0.74 J/g). The two different T_m indicates the presence of two thermal domains, likely caused by the melting and separation of myosin and actin components (Table 4. and Figure 4.) [23].

Discussion

Here we have shown that the thermal analyzes by differential scanning calorimetry clearly demonstrate significant differences between the pathologic and healthy groups, indicating that the thermal stability and protein conformation of the examined degenerative, ischemic or inflamed pathologic samples are significantly different from the intact tissue samples.

We have demonstrated a significant difference between the examined intact and ruptured tendons or degenerated joint capsules. The significant reduction in enthalpy is likely due to depolymerisation and denaturation of the collagen fibers. It is possible, that the overextension may result in an intermolecular and intrafibrillar sliding of the collagen. The collagen components then became re-organized, parallel with an increase of the level of type III collagen [24]. Therefore, the injured tissue became less compacted and cooperative, resulting in the overall decrease of the thermal enthalpy [4]. Taken together, the changes of thermal characteristics could be explained by the structural changes of the degenerated collagen (irregularity, scars), as a result of micro traumas and degeneration [5].

Recently, Chaudhury et al., has published data about the changes of thermal properties after human rotator cuff injuries. Consistently with our data, they found that the small and massive rotator cuff tears had significantly lower T_{onset}, T_{peak}, and ΔH (~4 J/g difference), compared to controls [25].

Meanwhile, the thermal enthalpy of the inflamed tissue samples was significantly increased, compared to the healthy origins. The chronic, non-specific inflammation may affect regulatory pathways interfering with extracellular matrix synthesis and inducing fibroblast proliferation. The production of irregular bundles and changes in the balance of different types of collagens could provide a possible explanation for the changes of the detected changes in the thermal characteristics [5, 8]. It is noteworthy, that both of cerebral palsy and the abnormal structural change of the muscle caused by clubfoot showed an increased global thermal stability, compared to the healthy controls. It could be caused by an impaired inter-domain communication of the different subunits of muscle proteins, resulting in muscle dysfunction or the different 'packaging' of the affected parts [9].

The compartment syndrome, which is an elevation of the interstitial pressure in closed fascial compartment, requires immediate surgical interventions. Therefore, it has a particular importance to differentiate accurately the affected components from the healthy parts [15, 26]. The DSC scans clearly demonstrated the significant differences between the different stages of compartment syndrome (Table 4.), supported by the calorimetric enthalpy values. These observations could be explained with the structural alterations caused by the biochemical processes and by the effect of compartmental pressure change.

Importantly, DSC could be a useful tool for determination of other human diseases. Könczöl F et al., has introduced DSC measurements for forensic investigation: in context with chemotherapy induced neuropathy, they found that the thermal denaturation of the affected muscle and nerve samples decreased, while the calorimetric enthalpy increased, depending on the therapeutic cyclophosphamide doses [27].

Table 4. The pressure and characteristic thermal parameters of intact and ischemic human skeletal muscle samples

		n	Compartment pressure	T_m (^{0}C)	ΔH_{cal} (J/g)
1	Healthy leg muscle	4	<30 mmHg	55.5 59.9	0.52 *
2	Compartment syndrome Gr. I. (mild)	4	30-35 mmHg	58.1 62.2	0.28 *
3	Compartment syndrome Gr. II. (severe)	4	>30 mmHg	57.45 61.5	0.24 *
4	Volkmann's ischemic contracture	3	N/A (chronic)	57.75 61.8 65.8	0.74 *

n: number of samples, T_m (^{0}C): melting temperature, ΔH_{cal} (J/g): calorimetric enthalpy. Unpaired Student's t-test, * indicates $p < 0.05$ vs. healthy collagen samples. Data are expressed as mean, $n \geq 3$ in each group.

Ischemia-reperfusion injury could also significantly affect the thermal characteristics of different tissue samples. Nedvig K et al., have recently demonstrated that DSC analyzes were helpful in the detection thermal characteristic changes of the small bowel structure, in a rabbit model of ischemia-reperfusion injury [28].

In New Zealand rabbit model of Staphylococcus aureus induced experimental septic knee joints arthritis, Sillinger et al., demonstrated that the development of infective structural destruction of the femoral cartilage could be confirmed by the means of DSC measurements [19]. Utilizing human tissue samples, Naumov et al., also found clear differences, comparing interfacial membranes collected after aseptic and septic loosening of hip prosthesis (aseptic membrane: $T_m = 62.2$ °C and $\Delta H_{cal} = 2.13$ J/g, septic membrane: $T_m = 60.2$ °C and $\Delta H_{cal} = 3.22$ J/g,) [18].

Conclusion

We have demonstrated a recognizable pattern in the thermal denaturation characteristics of the intra-operatively collected pathologic and healthy human tissue samples. Therefore, differential scanning calorimetry could provide clinically relevant information to achieve a more accurate intra-operative diagnosis and prognostic grading of different types of musculoskeletal diseases.

Acknowledgments

The SETARAM Micro DSC-II was purchased with a grant (CO-272) from the Hungarian Scientific Research Fund (Dénes Lőrinczy).

References

[1] Than, P; Domán, I; Lőrinczy, D. Differential scanning calorimetry in the research of degenerative musculoskeletal disorders. *Thermochimica Acta*, 2004, 415, 83-87.

[2] Charlson, ME; Allegrante, JP. Disparities in the use of total joint arthroplasty. *N Engl J Med*, 2000, 342, 1044-5.

[3] Amlang, MH; Zwipp, H. [Damage to large tendons: Achilles, patellar and quadriceps tendons]. *Chirurg*, 2006, 77, 637-649, quiz 649.

[4] Wiegand, N; Vámhidy, L; Lőrinczy, D. Differential scanning calorimetric examination of ruptured lower limb tendons in human. *Journal of Thermal Analysis and Calorimetry*, 2010, 101, 487-492.

[5] Wiegand, N; Vámhidy, L; Patczai, B; Dömse, E; Than, P; Kereskai, L; Lőrinczy, D. Differential scanning calorimetric examination of the degenerated human palmar aponeurosis in dupuytren disease. *Journal of Thermal Analysis and Calorimetry*, 2009, 95, 797-800.

[6] Clayton, RA; Court-Brown, CM. The epidemiology of musculoskeletal tendinous and ligamentous injuries. *Injury*, 2008, 39, 1338-44.

[7] Resch, H; Breitfuss, H. [Spontaneous tendon ruptures. Etiology, pathogenesis and therapy]. *Orthopade*, 1995, 24, 209-219.

[8] Wiegand, N; Vámhidy, L; Patczai, B; Dömse, E; Than, P; Kereskai, L; Lőrinczy, D. Differential scanning calorimetric examination of transverse carpal ligament in carpal tunnel disease. *Journal of Thermal Analysis and Calorimetry*, 2009, 95, 793-796.

[9] Gazso, I; Kránicz, J; Bellyei, Á; Lőrinczy, D. DSC analysis of the abnormalities of human leg skeletal muscles: A preliminary study. *Thermochimica Acta*, 2003, 402, 117-122.

[10] Wunderlich, B. Thermal analysis of macromolecules. *Journal of Thermal Analysis and Calorimetry*, 1996, 46, 643-679.

[11] Miles, CA; Burjanadze, TV; Bailey, AJ. The kinetics of the thermal denaturation of collagen in unrestrained rat tail tendon determined by differential scanning calorimetry. *J Mol Biol*, 1995, 245, 437-446.

[12] Comerford, EJ; Innes, JF; Tarlton, JF; Bailey, AJ. Investigation of the composition, turnover, and thermal properties of ruptured cranial cruciate ligaments of dogs. *Am J Vet Res*, 2004, 65, 1136-1141.

[13] Willett, TL; Labow, RS; Lee, JM. Mechanical overload decreases the thermal stability of collagen in an in vitro tensile overload tendon model. *J Orthop Res*, 2008, 26, 1605- 1610.

[14] Naumov, I; Wiegand, N; Patczai, B; Vámhidy, L; Lőrinczy D. Differential scanning calorimetric examination of the human hyaline cartilage of the femoral head after femoral neck fracture. *Journal of Thermal Analysis and Calorimetry*, 2012, 108, 59-65.

[15] Wiegand, N; Vámhidy, L; Patczai, B; Dömse, E; Kereskai, L; Lőrinczy, D. Differential scanning calorimetric examination of the human skeletal muscle in a compartment syndrome of the lower extremities. *Journal of Thermal Analysis and Calorimetry*, 2009, 98, 177-182.

[16] Doman, I; Illes, T; Lőrinczy, D. Differential sacnning calorimetric examination of the human intervertebral disc: establishment of calorimetric standards of different stages of degeneration. *Thermochimica Acta*, 2003, 405, 293-299.

[17] Bálint, G; Than, P; Domán, I; Wiegand, N; Horváth, G; Lőrinczy D. Calorimetric examination of the human meniscus. *Journal of Thermal Analysis and Calorimetry*, 2009, 95, 759-761.

[18] Naumov, I; Lőrinczy, D; Vámhidy, L; Than, P; Wiegand, N. Differential scanning calorimetric examination of the interfacial membrane in failed hip joint replacements. *Journal of Thermal Analysis and Calorimetry*, 2012, 109, 783-787.

[19] Sillinger, T; Than, P; Kocsis, B; Lőrinczy D. DSC measurement of cartilage destruction caused by septic arthritis. *Journal of Thermal Analysis and Calorimetry*, 2005, 82, 221-223.

[20] Bognár, G; Szabó, I; Bálint, L; Hepp, B; Kereskai, L; Lőrinczy D. Thermal effects of shoulder electrothermal arthroscopic capsulorrhaphy monitored by differential scanning calorimetry - A preliminary study. *Thermochimica Acta*, 2007, 464, 78-82.

[21] Wiegand, N; Naumov, I; Nöt, LG; Vámhidy, L; Lőrinczy D. Differential scanning calorimetric examination of pathologic scar tissues of human skin. *Journal of Thermal Analysis and Calorimetry*, 2013, 111, 1897-1902.

[22] Nöt, LG; Naumov, I; Vámhidy, L; Lőrinczy, D; Wiegand, N. Comparison of thermal characteristics of degenerated and inflamed human collagen structures with differential scanning calorimetry. *Journal of Thermal Analysis and Calorimetry*, 2013, 113, 273-279.

[23] Lőrinczy, D; Vértes, Z; Könczöl, F; Belágyi, J. Thermal transitions of actin. *Journal of Thermal Analysis and Calorimetry*, 2009, 95, 713-719.

[24] Eriksen, HA; Pajala, A; Leppilahti, J; Risteli, J. Increased content of type III collagen at the rupture site of human Achilles tendon. *J Orthop Res*, 2002, 20, 1352-1357.

[25] Chaudhury, S; Holland, C; Porter, D; Tirlapur, UK; Vollrath, F; Carr, AJ. Torn human rotator cuff tendons have reduced collagen thermal properties on differential scanning calorimetry. *J Orthop Res*, 2011, 29, 1938-1943.

[26] Bourne, RB; Rorabeck, CH. Compartment syndromes of the lower leg. *Clin Orthop Relat Res*, 1989, 240, 97-104.

[27] Könczöl, F; Wiegand, N; Nöt, LG; Lőrinczy, D. Examination of the cyclophosphamide-induced polyneuropathy on guinea pig sciatic nerve

and gastrocnemius muscle with differential scanning calorimetry. *Journal of Thermal Analysis and Calorimetry*, 2014, 115, 2239-43.

[28] Nedvig, K; Ferencz, A; Rőth, E; Lőrinczy D. DSC examination of intestinal tissue following warm ischemia and reperfusion injury. *Journal of Thermal Analysis and Calorimetry*, 2009, 95, 775-779.

In: Musculoskeletal Diseases
Editor: Greg Reed
ISBN: 978-1-63463-551-6

Chapter III

Effects of Stretching and Sensory Motor Training for Older Adults with Musculoskeletal Diseases

***Silvia Regina Valderramas*[1,3], *Elisangela Valevein Rodrigues*[2,4], *Talita Gianello Gnoato Zotz*[2], *Luiza Herminia Gallo*[2] and *Anna Raquel Silveira Gomes*[1,2]**

[1]Physiotherapy Department,
Federal University of Parana (UFPR), Brazil
[2]Physical Education Postgraduate Program,
Federal University of Parana (UFPR), Brazil
[3]Medicina Interna Postgraduate Program,
Federal University of Parana (UFPR), Brazil
[4]Federal Institute of Parana (IFPR), Curitiba, Parana, Brazil

Abstract

The ageing process is responsible per se for a series of morphological and functional alterations of the musculoskeletal system, which can compromise the functional independence of the elderly. It is common the decrease in muscle mass (sarcopenia) and in muscle force (dinapenia). It also occurs increase in the stiffness of the muscle-tendon unit, decrease in fascicle length and in the pennation angle related to the aged. These changes negatively affect the muscle strength and may also impair the mobility, balance and gait of the older adults. When associated with physical inactivity there is a potentiation of the deleterious effects resulted from aging process, and these situations can be recognized as musculoskeletal diseases. Still, the poor mobility associated with decrease in muscle strength and balance can increase the chances of falls in this population. Thus, to mitigate and/or reverse these changes it has been recommended regular physical activity and//or systematic exercise. A number of different types of exercise have been suggested, among them stretching, neuromotor and balance exercises are emphasized. Stretching exercises, when performed by a period equal to or greater than four weeks with three to four repetitions and duration between 30 and 60 seconds, has proved to be effective not only in improving flexibility and range of motion, but also gait speed, which is related with a lower risk of falls. Among the neuromotor exercises, video game exercise training has been shown to be effective in improving balance, agility and muscular strength, and also in reducing the risk of falls in community elderly. For a specific balance training, it has been recommended that this must be composed by gradual exercise in complexity and support base, starting from simple postures and greater support and developing throughout training; dynamic movements that can alter the center of gravity, recruiting postural muscles; and can also reduce the sensory imput information, for example, perform the same exercise, but with eyes closed. The training should be performed two to three times a week, lasting 20-30 minutes per session. Thus, it is emphasized the importance of exercise for older people, especially regular stretching, balance and neuromotor ones can be adopted to prevent and/or improve flexibility, balance, mobility, comorbidities and musculoskeletal diseases in this population.

Introduction

Ageing is a highly complex, dynamic and irreversible process, associated with the deterioration and restructuring of the functions of the entire human body, the systems which most suffer the effects of this process being the nervous, endocrine, immune and musculoskeletal systems (Rocha, Reis, Teixeira, 2010).

Musculoskeletal ageing negatively affects muscle mass and strength, balance and various functional abilities (Ballak et al., 2014). When associated with physical inactivity or bedridden and/or immobilization periods, there is a potentiation of the deleterious effects resulting from the aging process, and these situations can be recognized as musculoskeletal diseases such as sarcopenia, dynapenia, cachexia and a set of changes together known as the fragility syndrome (Ballak et al., 2014; Cruz-Jentoft et al., 2010; Hall et al., 2011). In addition, the poor mobility associated with the decrease in muscle strength and balance can increase the chances of falls in older people (Melzer et al., 2004; Ruwer et al., 2005; Lang et al., 2010). It is estimated that about 30% of elderly people over 65, and 50% of the over 80s fall at least once a year, and the main result of this has been hip fractures, and in 25% of the cases of fracture, in death (Melzer et al., 2004).

Thus, regular physical activity and/or systematic exercises have been recommended to mitigate and/or reverse these changes (Garber et al., 2011). A number of different types of exercise have been suggested, amongst which stretching, motor neuron and balance exercises are emphasized, which could be adopted to prevent and/or improve flexibility, balance, mobility, comorbidities and musculoskeletal diseases in this population (Garber et al., 2011).

In this chapter the principal musculoskeletal changes associated with the ageing process, the main musculoskeletal diseases currently appearing in the elderly and the prescription of stretching, balance and sensory motor exercises for this population, will be presented.

1. Musculoskeletal Changes Associated with the Ageing Process

1.1. Ageing of the Extracellular Matrix (ECM)

The ageing process deteriorates the mechanical properties of muscle tissue, which contributes to a loss of function and independence by the elderly (Trappe, 2009). Such a deterioration of the mechanical properties of the muscle is attributed to a reduction in muscle mass and contractile proteins. In addition the loss in muscle strength together with the reduction in muscle mass and changes in the ECM, also contribute to the declining process of the mechanical properties (Trappe, 2009; Narici & Maffulli, 2010; Kragstrup, Kjaer, Mackey, 2011).

The structural, biochemical and cellular changes in the extracellular matrix (ECM) lead to an increase in muscle rigidity and consequent reduction in function with ageing. The concentrations of collagen, of enzymatic mediators of the collagen cross-links and of the final products of advanced glycation (AGE), appear to lead to an increase in collagen deposition in ageing muscle. These concentrations are also related to alterations in the proportions of collagen types I and III in ageing muscle (Kragstrup, Kjaer & Mackey, 2011; Mattiello-Sverzut et al., 2013). In addition ECM ageing is associated with alteration in mechanotransduction, reduction in satellite cell activation and retardation of inflammatory chemotactic responses (Kragstrup, Kjaer & Mackey, 2011). Figure 1 exemplifies the ageing mechanism in skeletal muscle ECM.

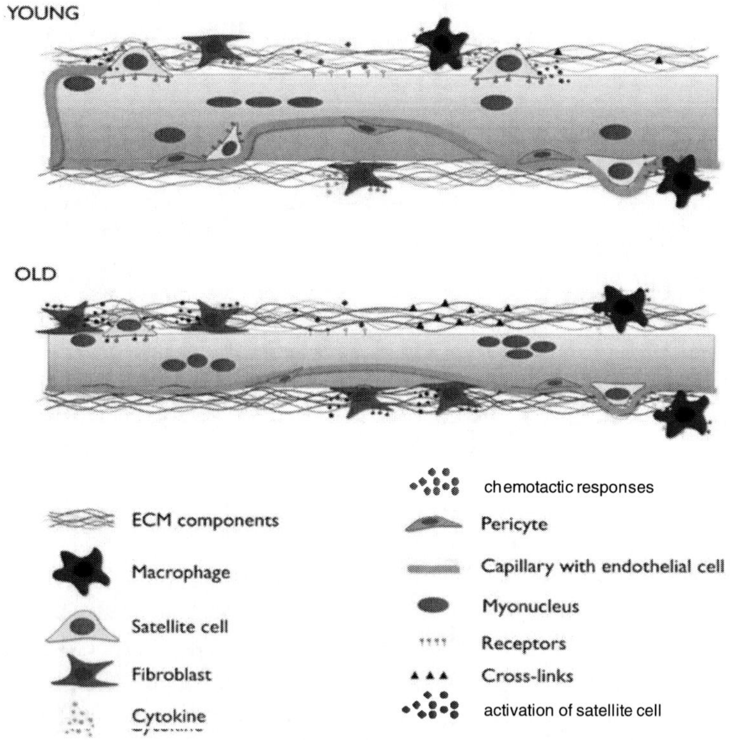

Figure 1. Illustration of the changes in skeletal muscle extracellular matrix (ECM), comparing the young with the old. Red lines represent collagen I deposition on the ECM and blue lines represent collagen III deposition on the ECM. Adapted from Kragstrup, Kjaer & Mackey (2011).

1.2. Functional Changes in the Skeletal Muscle

Apart from the decrease in muscle mass, changes in the muscle architecture and tendon properties also occur, with repercussions on muscle function (Narici et al., 2007). When compared with younger individuals, elderly men and women show less tendon rigidity, stress and tension, and decreases in the cross-sectional area, in muscle thickness, in the length of the fascia and in the pennation angle (Carrol et al., 2008; Couppé et al., 2009; Fukumoto et al., 2012; Stenroth et al., 2012; Baroni et al., 2013).

On comparing young and elderly individuals with the same level of physical activity, a reduction of from 30 to 60% in the maximum strength of the knee extensor muscles was observed (Baroni et al., 2013). Ageing brings an even greater decline in muscle power (3-4% per year) when compared with maximum muscle strength (1-2% per year) (Izquierdo et al., 1999; Skelton et al., 1994). Specifically with respect to the quadriceps muscles, individuals aged ~75 years old presented only 62.2% of the ability to generate strength when compared with young adults (36.5 years old) (Frontera et al., 2000).

Such changes can directly influence muscle function, since there is a relationship between the mechanical properties of the tendon and its capacity to produce muscle strength (Stenroth et al., 2012). Changes in the length of the fascia can also alter the optimum angle for strength production, making the speed of muscle contraction slower (Lieber et al., 2000).

The age related decline in muscle capacity especially affects the ankle plantar flexor muscles, which are important during locomotion, such that compensatory actions are necessary such as a decrease in step length and a change in the kinetic moment of strength of the ankle, knees and hips (Kulmala et al., 2014). In fact, Kulmala et al., (2014) observed a 22% decrease in the generation of power by the ankle when compared to the younger group, and an increase in the knee flexion angle and in the eccentric power, with a tendency for greater hip flexion. The compensatory action causes an alteration in the ankle kinetics when walking, and with this the elderly use the ankle flexor muscles less and the knee and hip joints more. Thus the capacity of the ankle flexor muscles to generate strength is highly important in the maintenance of locomotive performance (De Vita, Hortobagyi, 2000; Monaco et al., 2009; Cofré et al., 2011; Boyer et al., 2012; Kulmala et al., 2014).

Body balance is directly affected by changes in the functions of the muscles involved in walking, especially those of the ankle, since this joint is amongst three movement strategies that can be used to return the body to a state of balance: Ankle strategy, knee strategy and take a step forward (Horak,

2006). Elderly individuals who fall over easily use the hip strategies and the step forward much more than those who do not fall over so easily, who trust in their ankle joints to maintain their balance (Makki, 2000).

Hasson et al., (2014) observed that the elderly showed worse postural performance in both static and dynamic activities, and that this result was strongly related to muscle strength. Balance also presented a relationship with other muscle parameters such as fiber length and muscle power (capacity to generate strength as a function of speed). In general, the muscle properties explained 50-60% of the alterations in balance, and the remaining alterations could be related to other factors such as the reaction time and sensory aspects (Lord et al., 1991; Hasson et al., 2014).

2. Main Musculoskeletal Diseases

2.1. Sarcopenia

Sarcopenia is a musculoskeletal disease characteristic of senescence, although it can occur without appearance of the latter, which can be accelerated as a result of some chronic diseases (Cruz-Jentoft et al., 2010). In addition, sarcopenia has an important correlation with posture and locomotion maintenance in the elderly and with the ability to carry out everyday activities (Thompson, 2002). The relative decrease in muscle mass occurs gradually over time, and appears to behave similarly for both men and women (Strugnell et al., 2014). Reports can be found in the literature of muscle mass reductions of 11.3% and 15.4% in men and women, respectively, between 25 and 91 years of age (Strugnell et al., 2014). The following table exemplifies the loss of muscle volume over a lifetime and its relationship with physical function. The table shows the relationship between the muscle compartments and the physical performance of younger and elderly adults (Buford et al., 2012). The muscle volume of the femoral region appears to be strongly associated with physical function in older adults (Buford et al., 2012).

According to Hall et al., (2011), sarcopenia is multifactorial and occurs as the result of the ageing process, where common questions related to ageing, such as: Reduction in amino acid absorption, which leads to a decrease in anabolic activity and consequent decrease in muscle mass, associated with a reduction in physical activity and motor neuron activity, contribute to muscle atrophy and consequently to sarcopenia.

Table 1. Skeletal muscle volume and functional aspects

	Anthropometrics characteristics; Skeletal Muscle Volume and functional aspects
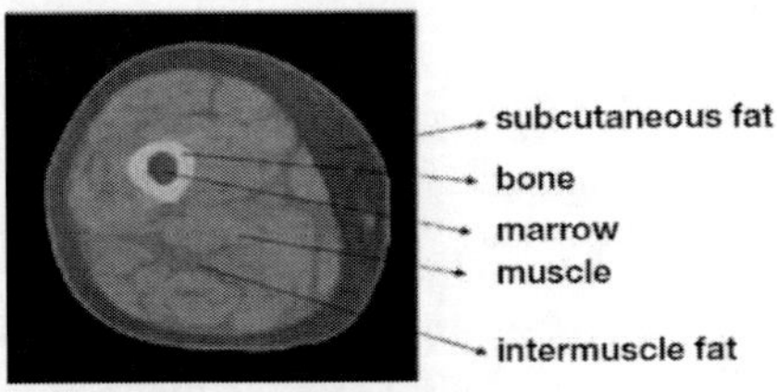	
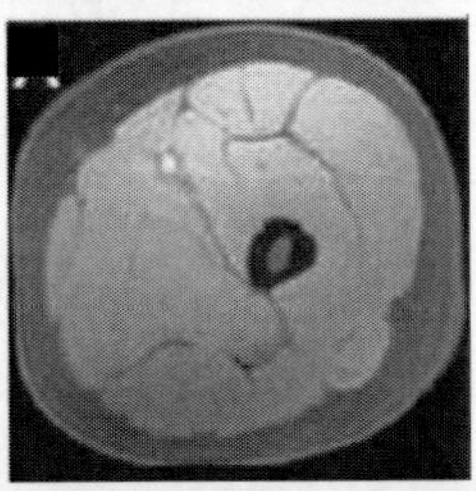	Age: 33 years old Gender: Male BMI: 24.5 kg/m2 Skeletal muscle volume: 588.5 cm3 Subcutaneous mass: 308.4 cm3 Intramuscular mass: 78.7 cm3
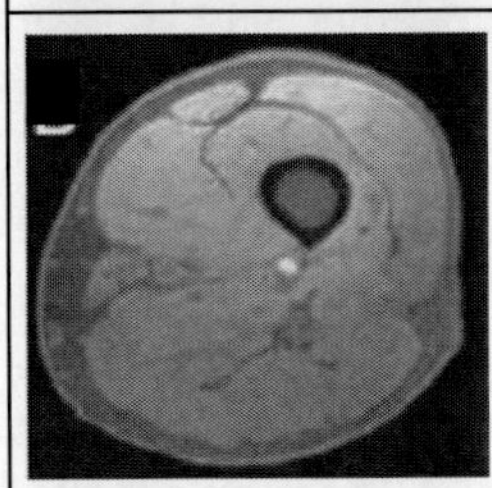	Age: 73 years old Gender: Male SPPB: 11 Gait speed: 1.15m/s BMI: 24.9 kg/m2 Skeletal muscle volume: 461.3 cm3 Subcutaneous mass: 194.7 cm3 Intramuscular mass: 113.8
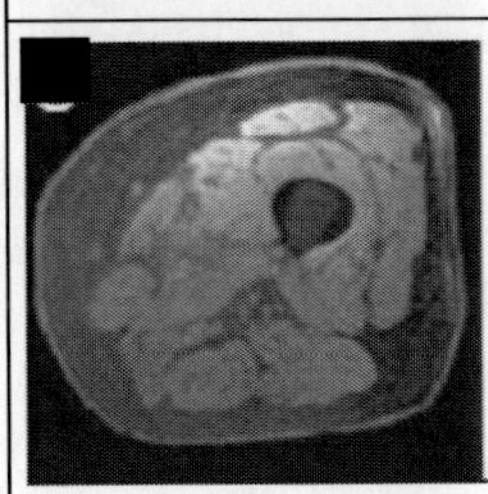	Age: 84 years old Gender: Male SPPB: 6 Gait speed: 0.49m/s BMI: 26.9 kg/m2 Skeletal muscle volume: 364.7 cm3 Subcutaneous mass: 339.3 Intramuscular mass: 131.7 cm3

Adapted from Buford et al., (2012). SPPB: Short Physical Performance Battery; BMI: body mass index.

It is known that this is related to alterations in the architecture of the skeletal muscle, such as: Reduction in muscle size, that is, the muscle fascicles decrease in length and the pennation angle also decreases (Narici et al., 2003; Morse et al., 2005); decrease in the cross-sectional area of the muscle fibers, especially of type IIA; infiltration of intra-muscle fat and of conjunctive tissue; alterations of the acting; reduction by 24-30% of the strong myosin head; decreases in the dihydropiridin (DHPR) and ryanodine (RyR) receptors, compromising the coupling-excitation-contraction mechanism, and a fall in the isokinetic peak torque (60°/s and 240°/s). The latter two aspects could explain the reduction in muscle power and motor slowdown in the elderly (Doherty, 2003; Frontera et al., 2008; Muscaritoli et al., 2010; Narici, Maganaris, 2007). However, the decline in muscle strength is quicker than the loss in muscle mass (Clark, Manini, 2010).

Sarcopenia is more accentuated in women as from middle age due to the menopause, which is associated with a decrease in female hormones which induces alterations in the skeletal muscle and bones (Dione, 2000; Cooper, 2008). With respect to muscle tissue, changes occur in the contractile properties due to a reduced capacity to synthesize new proteins, the resulting imbalance between muscle protein synthesis and degradation, the increase in conjunctive tissue and intramuscular fat, the decrease in the muscle fiber cross-sectional area and decrease in the number of muscle estrogen receptors (Kadi et al., 2002; Maltais et al., 2009).

Some studies have reported that sarcopenia could be associated with the frailty syndrome, whose consequences are: Decrease in muscle strength, low tolerance to exercise and a reduction in walking speed (Macedo, Gazzola & Najas, 2008; Walston et al., 2006). In addition Walston et al., (2006) reported that sarcopenia consisted of multiple mechanisms involving as from the systematic and organic cell-molecular level: Oxidative damage to the mitochondrial DNA, cell senescence, hormonal dysregulation and malnutrition. It is important to emphasize that sarcopenia is distinct from the cachexia caused by inflammatory diseases, advanced chronic diseases, debilitating muscle diseases or malnutrition (Doherty, 2003; Roubenoff et al., 1997). In these situations there is a reduction in skeletal muscle mass (sarcopenia), which is just one of the clinical manifestations of the more complex syndromes known as cachexia.

2.2. Dynapenia

The reduction in muscle strength characteristic of the ageing process is known as dynapenia (Clark & Manini, 2008). According to Clark & Manini

(2008), the concept of dynapenia was created to differentiate the loss of muscle mass from the loss of muscle strength, since the loss of muscle mass (sarcopenia) on its own does not explain the loss of muscle strength (dynapenia). The loss of muscle strength and power which occurs with increasing age is related to myogenic and neural factors, and is strongly correlated with the risk of falls (Lord et al., 2002; Pijnappels et al., 2008). The preferential atrophy of type II muscle fibers, motoneuron denervation, greater co-activation of the antagonistic musculature and a decrease in the levels of physical activity in the aged are some of the causes of dynapenia (Miszko et al., 2003).

2.3. Cachexia

Cachexia is a fatal syndrome (Dodson et al., 2010; Hall et al., 2011), characterized by rapid muscle atrophy, leading to a reduction in motor function (Palus et al., 2014). It has been estimated that 40% of the patients with chronic conditions such as: Chronic obstructive pulmonary disease (COPD), cardiac, renal and hepatic insufficiencies, cancer, AIDS and sepsis, suffer from cachexia (Ali & Garcia, 2014).

Resulting from disease-induced physiological changes (Ali & Garcia, 2014; Palus et al., 2014), the inflammatory cytokines have a fundamental role in the induction of sarcopenia and cachexia, acute inflammatory processes resulting from diseases inducing cachexia, and chronic inflammatory processes resulting from the ageing process, leading to sarcopenia (Hall et al., 2011; Palus et al., 2014). Thus cachexia can induce sarcopenia but the contrary does not occur (Hall et al., 2011).

Cachexia is a complex, multifactorial syndrome characterized by weight loss, predominantly a loss of body mass and adipose tissue (Ali & Garcia, 2014), anorexia, hypoalbuminemia, anemia, changes in wound healing and in immunocompetence (Rocha et al., 2010). It presents changes such as a reduction in the basal metabolic rate, and the functioning of the upper and lower limbs, which start to become slower. In addition motor function is prejudiced and the psychological stress causes a loss of appetite, and difficulties in chewing and swallowing. This group of dysfunctions leads to a degeneration in health of the elderly person and can consequently lead to death (Sperotto & Spinelli, 2010).

At the Cachexia Consensus Conference in 2006, the condition was defined as the presence of chronic disease and a weight loss of $\geq$ 5% in a period of less than 12 months or a BMI below 20 kg/m^2, associated with at least three of the following criteria: 1) decrease in muscle strength, 2) fatigue, 3) anorexia, 4) reduction in the fat-free mass index and 5) biochemical abnormalities such as inflammation, anemia or a reduction in the serum albumin concentration. Another point to be highlighted is the difference between cachexia and malnutrition states or anorexia. The latter are conditions that can be reversed with adequate food ingestion, a situation difficult to occur with cachexia (Evans et al., 2006).

2.4. Frailty Syndrome

Frailty is a multifactorial geriatric condition known for more than 30 years, but still without a universally accepted definition due to its physical-pathological complexity (Moretto et al., 2012). In general it is characterized by a decline in energy reserves, neuroendocrine dysregulation, a lowering of the immune function and a reduction in resistance to stressors, resulting from senescence and interaction with current and accumulated health and functionality risks (Fried et al., 2001; Neri et al., 2013).

The frail aged make up a subgroup of individuals susceptible to adverse health outcomes such as incapacity, hospitalization and death, due to a reduction in their response to stressful conditions, a vulnerability which predisposes them to chronic diseases, anorexia, sarcopenia, osteopenia, cognitive deficits and incapacity (Ferrucci et al., 2004; Neri et al., 2013).

In an epidemiological study with 65 to 79 year old frail women, a relationship between their frailty and ischemic heart disease, encephalic vascular accident (EVA), COPD, *diabetes mellitus* (DM), high blood pressure and osteoarthritis was evident. The prevalence of physical incapacities was greater amongst the frail women when compared with non-frail women. An increasing risk for frailty associated positively with a low socioeconomic level, a history of ischemic heart disease, DM. hip fractures, COPD, osteoarthritis, EVA and depression (Ferrucci et al., 2004).

Starting with the sub-clinical phase (pre-fragile condition), the process can evolve without much temporal precision to clinical manifestations, and the greatest potential for prevention is in the stage anteceding these manifestations. After installation of the phenomenon, the objective of therapeutic treatment is to prevent, postpone or soothe the adverse effects (Teixeira & Neri, 2006).

Table 2. Reference values for grip strength, stratified by gender and body mass index (BMI)

Men		Women	
BMI (kg/m²)	Strength (kgF)	BMI (kg/m²)	Strength (kgF)
≤ 24	≤ 29	≤ 23	≤ 17
24.1-26	≤ 30	23.1-26	≤ 17.3
26.1-28	≤ 30	26.1-29	≤ 18.3
> 28	≤ 32	> 29	≤ 21

Based on Fried et al., (2001).

Table 3. Reference values for walk time, stratified by gender and height

Men		Women	
Height	Time	Height	Time
≤ 173 cm	≥ 7 seconds	≤ 159 cm	≥ 7 seconds
> 173 cm	≥ 6 seconds	> 159 cm	≥ 6 seconds

Based on Fried et al., (2001).

To evaluate the syndrome, Fried et al., (2001) proposed a model for the frail phenotype, composed of the evaluation of five items: 1) non-intentional weight loss in the previous year above 4.5 kg or 5% of the body weight; 2) Auto-reported fatigue, evaluated from two questions found on the CES-D Depression Scale (Center for Epidemiological Studies) - with respect to the previous week ask the elderly person is asked the frequency with which he/she had to make an effort to carry out habitual tasks, and if he/she did not manage to carry out his/her activities: Rarely or none of the time - 1 day (0); some or a little of the time - 1-2 days (1); a moderate amount of the time - 3-4 days (2); or most of the time (3). If the participant reported 2 or 3, the value was considered for scoring; 3) decrease in hand gripping strength measured with a dynamometer and with reference values adjusted for gender and body mass index (BMI) - Table 2, 4) self-report of a low level of physical activity evaluated using the short version of the Minnesota questionnaire, which provides values of the weekly energy expenditure in kcal of the physical activities and exercises, adjusted according to gender: Men < 383 and women < 270 kcal physical activity/ week are frail; 5) low walking speed in seconds, with reference values adjusted according to gender and height for walking a distance of 4.5 m - Table 3.

The classification is made according to the quantity of factors the person presents: No factor is considered robust, from one to two factors - pre-frail and with a high risk of developing the syndrome, and three or more factors - frail (Fried et al., 2001; Macedo, Gazzola & Najas, 2008). In this way the phenotype would be the result of one cycle, in which the start is still not clearly specified. The cycle is represented by a spiral with decreasing multiple system energy reserve potential, and hypothetically explains the conditions of fatigue, weight loss and alterations in walking speed, justifying the high risk for the adverse consequences of the syndrome (Figure 2).

It is also important to consider that frailty, since it is a multifactorial and dynamic syndrome, is inserted in a context that involves social, clinical, cognitive, psychological and environmental factors, in addition to biological factors, throughout the lifetime (Bergman et al., 2004). Thus, apart from the phenotype proposed by Fried et al., (2001), there is also the Edmonton Scale for the evaluation of frailty, which evaluates other domains: Cognitive, functional independence, social support, use of medication, nutrition, humor, continence and functional performance; and classifies the elderly person as: Apparently vulnerable, slightly frail, moderately frail and severely frail (Teixeira, 2006).

2.5. Osteoarthritis

One of the consequences of an ageing population is the increase in chronic-degenerative diseases, amongst which osteoarthritis (OA) is the most prevalent joint disease amongst the elderly population, causing a socioeconomic impact due to the incapacities appearing in the individuals (Petrella et al., 2012).

OA is a degenerative disease characterized by the progressive loss of cartilage (van Leeuwen et al., 2014), its presence in the lower limbs being the greatest cause of disability, injuries and dependence in the elderly, shown to have difficulty in carrying out the everyday activities, particularly in mobility and transference tasks, favoring a risk of falls and worsening the quality of life of this population (Sturnieks, et al., 2004; Petrella et al., 2012; Khalaj et al., 2014; Larmer et al., 2014).

The risk factors for OA include ageing, sex, genetic factors, occupational factors, previous injuries and obesity (Larmer et al., 2014). The elderly with OA in their lower limbs show a greater risk of falls due to failures in the neuromuscular systems, such as reduced levels of muscle strength (Borin et al., 2010; Larmer et al., 2014; Mat et al., 2014). A strength deficit in the quadriceps of between 20% and 70% stands out in individuals with OA in the knees, and of between 20% and 31% in the periarticular muscles in those with OA in the hips.

Proprioceptive deficits are also common in arthritic populations, and altered sensory information as from the joint surfaces, capsule and ligaments of arthritic joints can result in prejudice in the perception of the positions of the limbs, necessary for safe movement (Sturnieks et al., 2004; Khalaj et al., 2014; Petrella et al., 2012). Summing these changes up together, OA causes a reduction in the amplitude of movement, contributing to a compromise in the semi-static and dynamic balances (Petrella et al., 2012).

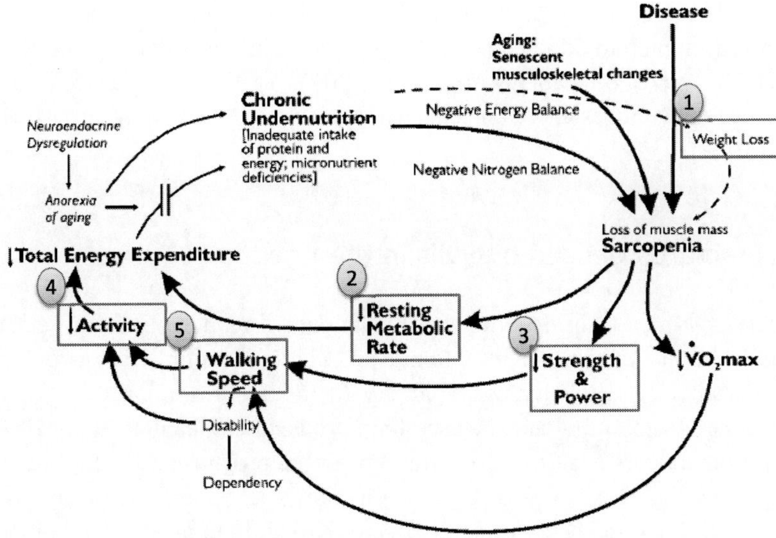

Figure 2. Cycle of frailty hypothesized as consistent with demonstrated pairwise associations and clinical signs and symptoms of frailty. Adapted from Fried & Walston, 2000.

In knees affected by advanced OA, the pain, inflammation and joint laxity also contribute to deficits in proprioception which alter the way of walking. As a response to this process, one can observe a decrease in the support time and increase in the risk of falls (Bacarin et al., 2004; Khalaj et al., 2014).

When conservative treatments of knee OA are ineffective, total knee arthroplasty (TKA) may be indicated, which can reduce the pain and improve the physical performance of these individuals (van Leeuwen et al., 2014).

TKA is considered to be the standard golden treatment for the final stages of knee OA (Pozzi, Snyder-Mackler, Zeni, 2013).

In elderly individuals submitted to total knee arthroplasty, in which the joint is reconstructed with the finality of restoring its movement and function, the musculoskeletal deficits, amongst which proprioception, are more significant, since they add to the age-related losses. A decrease in knee proprioception could be related to the removal of structures that contain mechanoreceptors during the surgery, such as: Joint capsule and the knee ligaments, principally the posterior cruciate ligament, and also the pain presented by knee OA, which compromises proprioception, inhibiting the peripheral reflexes (Bacarin et al., 2004; Ribeiro, Oliveira, 2008).

Another problem that should be taken into consideration is the considerable decrease in strength of the quadriceps immediately after TKA, which is attributed to deficits in activation and to muscle atrophy (Petterson et al., 2009; Pozzi, Snyder-Mackler, Zeni, 2013), which may be related to functional deficiencies and biomechanical asymmetry (Pozzi, Snyder-Mackler, Zeni, 2013).

2.6. Fractures Caused by Falls in the Aged

The post-menopausal period or involutional osteoporosis in the elderly affect the frailty of the proximal femur and can lead to hip fractures. Three methods are of great value to avoid hip fractures: Prevention of falls, the treatment of osteoporosis and the use of hip protectors (Sakamoto et al., 2006).

Various factors exist that affect the functional prognosis after hip fracture surgery, such as: Decrease in physical function; the occurrence of new falls and fractures, and the need for support care (Kronborg et al., 2014). Although the patients follow a post-surgery exercise program, a reduction of more than 50% in knee extension strength of the fractured limb in relation to the non-fractured one can be observed during the first week after hip surgery, prejudicing physical function (Kronborg et al., 2014).

Rehabilitation of individuals with hip fractures should be based on a multidisciplinary team, with psychological treatment to reduce anxiety, orientation about the surgery and post-operative phase, muscle strengthening of the upper limbs, especially the hip abductors, maintenance of the hip movement amplitude, respiratory exercises to prevent respiratory complications, orientation concerning the position in bed: Such as getting up and lying down, changes in lying down, how to use the toilet, wheelchair and frame (Donohue et al., 2013; Wilson, 2013).

2.6.1. Factors Related to Falls in the Elderly

Approximately one third of the elderly who live in communities fall at least once a year in developed countries, the incidence increasing with age. The falls occur in approximately 50% of the elderly over 85 years in age, with a profound impact on their health and quality of life (Segev-Jacubovski et al., 2011).

It can be seen that between 5 and 10% of the falls result in serious injury, such as head injuries or fractures. Even in the absence of a history of falls or when the fall caused no physical damage, about one third of the elderly develop a fear of falling which leads to self-imposed restrictions in mobility, reduced activity, depression and social isolation, with a subsequent increase in the risk of falls. It is therefore not surprising that the falls and injuries caused by the falls are of great concern to health professionals, since they represent an enormous problem for the individuals, for society and for the health systems. In 2008, the costs related to fatal and non-fatal falls were estimated at US$23.3 billion in the USA and US$1.6 billion just in the United Kingdom (Segev-Jacubovski et al., 2011).

It is well established that falls are a serious socioeconomic problem, with an annual cost of about 1% of the total national health costs (Segev-Jacubovski et al., 2011; König et al., 2014).

The causes of falls in the elderly are considered to be multifactorial, related to intrinsic and extrinsic factors. The intrinsic factors are characterized by declines in the following: Sensory-motor, visual, postural stability, balance, vestibular function, cognition, pain, psychological aspects such as a fear of falling and depression, changes in walking patterns, and the use of psychotropic medication (Pijnappels et al., 2008; Callisaya et al., 2009; Guimarães, Farinatti, 2005; Melzer et al., 2004; Chen et al., 1996; Leonard et al., 1997; Delbaere et al., 2009; Iinattiniemi et al., 2009). The extrinsic factors are characterized by social and environmental aspects (slippery surfaces, mats or loose floorboards, inadequate lighting, objects strewn on the floor, stairs without handrails and loose animals) (Clemson et al., 2008). The risk of falling increases according to the number of risk factors present and with age (Linattiniemi et al., 2009).

Studies have indicated that female sex, decrease in stature with advancing age, low body weight, central obesity, frailty, polypharmacy and pre-prandial hyperglycemia are factors associated with falls in elderly community dwellers

(Wu et al., 2013), as also a low educational level, greater body mass index (BMI), small family income, difficulty in using public transport, the use of walking aids (walking sticks, frames), limited perception of physical health, self-reported balance problems and an inability to get up from a chair at knee height (Kumar et al., 2014).

Table 4. Summary of age-related factors associated with falls

Intrinsic	Extrinsic
Compromising of the sensory-motor system: Visual, vestibular & proprioceptive	Social aspects: Small Family income Difficulty in using public transport Low educational level
Musculoskeletal modifications: decrease in muscle mass	Environmental factors:
Compromising of the cardiovascular system	Shoe type (high heels, use socks to walk about at home)
Slower postural responses	Loose carpets or floorboards
Cognitive changes and depression	Inadequate lighting
Decrease in postural control	Slippery floor surfaces
Neuromuscular diseases: Parkinson, Strokes	Objects scattered on the floor
Use of psychotropic medication and/or a combination of various medications (polypharmacy)	Stairs with no handrail
Diabetes	Loose animals
Use of orthoses	
Low health self-perception	

The methods normally used to check the risk of falls are: Self-applied questionnaires and clinical, laboratory and functional mobility evaluations (König et al., 2014).

Independent of the tools used to investigate the mechanisms involved in falls, the best predictor of independence, as also the factor most used to forecast falls, is the history of falls. The relative risk of an aged individual suffering a fall is about three times greater for individuals who already suffered a fall than for those who never did. Although the addition of the history of falls can improve the precision and reliability in the identification of individuals with a high risk for falls, it is also important to identify individuals with an imminent risk for a first time fall (König et al., 2014).

The multifactorial nature of falls and the lack of a strong fall-related biomarker make the identification of first-time fallers an increasing challenge (König et al., 2014). Mean walking parameters and their variability are key components in the evaluation of motor deficits related to falls in the aged, and can help clinical screening programs to identify first-time fallers (König et al., 2014).

Approximately 30% of the aged present walking disorders which could be associated with a reduction in independence, falls, hospitalization, institutionalization and mortality (Callisaya et al., 2009).

Visual difficulties result in changes in the processing of information, leading to spatial imprecision, making it more difficult to surmount obstacles and maintain postural control. Vestibular hypofunction leads to changes in walking mode and includes postural instability, wide-based walking and instability on curves, which can increase the risk of falls (Rogers, 2010).

A structured physical exercise program is indicated to prevent falls in the aged. This chapter will include stretching exercises and sensory motor training aimed at preventing falls in the aged, as also the prescription of exercises for individuals with osteoarthritis.

3. Stretching Exercise Prescription for Older Adults

In addition to the age-related musculoskeletal changes already dealt with in this chapter, joint mobility stands out, which can affect the levels of flexibility (Garber, 2011; Gallon et al., 2011). It appears that the decrease in flexibility does not occur with the same magnitude for all the body joints (Doriot, Wang, 2006; Soucie et al., 2010). Soucie et al., (2010) compared movement amplitudes for different age ranges, for both sexes. On comparing the age range of 20-44 and 45-69 for the female sex, the authors found significant reductions of: 7.73% for hip extension, 15.9% for dorsiflexion, 9.0% for ankle plantar flexion and 23.4% for elbow extension. When the comparison was made between the sexes, women presented greater movement amplitudes for ankle plantar flexion and for elbow pronation and supination than men for all the age ranges evaluated. Thus independent of the magnitude of the alterations observed for the different joint movements evaluated, women seem to maintain greater flexibility scores with the advance of age than men.

With a view to attenuating and/or improvement of the flexibility scores, the inclusion of stretching routines in training programs has been recommended, especially when directed at the elderly population (Garber, 2011). The effects promoted by muscle stretching exercises can be divided into acute and chronic ones. The effects of stretching are considered to be acute when the results are immediate and short term, lasting for seconds, minutes or hours after intervention (Taylor et al., 1990; Shier, 2004; Ryan et al., 2008; Weppler & Magnusson, 2010) or up to one week (Kamikawa et al., 2013). In this case the stretching exercise promotes an increase in length of the muscle-tendon unit of the ROM and improves tolerance to stretching (Kokkonen et al., 1998, Nelson et al., 2005; Kokkonen et al., 2007, Baranda & Ayala, 2010).

On the other hand the chronic effects represent the delayed results of stretching which can last for days, weeks or months (Gajdosik et al., 2005; Weppler & Magnusson, 2010). The following chronic effects were verified in rats: An increase in the serial sarcomere number, muscle fiber hypertrophy and molecular reorganization of the collagen bundles in the rat soleus (Coutinho et al., 2004; Coutinho et al., 2006; Secchi et al., 2008).

With respect to the chronic effects resulting from regular practice of stretching exercises in humans, gains in joint movement amplitude, muscle-tendon length and flexibility (Feland et al., 2001; Stanziano et al., 2009; Gallon et al., 2011; Costa et al., 2013); improvements in walking parameters (Christiansen et al., 2008; Cristopolisk et al., 2009; Kerrigan et al., 2003); improvements in muscle strength/torque, functionality and balance (Gajdosik et al., 2005a; Stanziano et al., 2009; Batista et al., 2009; Locks et al., 2012); improvements in agility and walking ability (Gajdosik et al., 2005a; Stanziano et al., 2009); and improvements in tolerance to stretching (Konrad & Tilp, 2014) have been observed.

In humans it was observed that stretching, when practiced every day for 6 weeks, did not alter the muscle architecture, that is, the length of the fascicles and muscle-tendon unit or the pennation angle, but increased the tolerance to stretching (Konrad & Tilp, 2014). In addition in a previous study, it was reported that when the gastrocnemius or anterior tibial muscles of humans were stretched when relaxed, more than half the change in muscle-tendon length was due to the tendon (Hoang et al., 2007). Still, in view of the literature searched, there is only one study that investigated the serial sarcomere number in humans, which found sarcomerogenesis one year after femoral lengthening, endorsing the capacity of human muscle to adapt to length modifications (Boakes et al., 2006).

Considering that some studies developed with rats did not find increase in the muscle length but verified addition in serial sarcomere number, after stretching protocols, it cannot be excluded the possibility of sarcomerogenesis in human, after a chronic training of flexibility (Secchi et al., 2008; Macedo et al., 2014; Weppler, Magnusson, 2010). Nevertheless, as the analysis of serial sarcomere number in human demand complex methods, ultrasound has become an important tool to evaluate the muscle architecture (Zöllner et al., 2012; Konrad & Tilp, 2014). For these motives it has been postulated that the chronic effects caused by the regular practice of stretching exercises in humans, could be caused by neural factors because it provokes an increase in stretching tolerance (Weppler, Magnusson, 2010; Konrad & Tilp, 2014).

Consensus has not yet been reached on the benefits of stretching exercises, be they acute or chronic, and there is much variation with respect to the parameters necessary for prescription, such as: Stretching technique used, time the stimulus is maintained for, number of repetitions, interval between repetitions, number of series, volume of training, daily and weekly frequency, and the specificity for each age range (Zotz et al., 2014). Table 5 presents the main studies that analyzed the chronic effects of stretching in the aged and their results.

Zotz et al., (2014) made a systematic review with a meta-analysis and verified that supervised static muscle stretching exercise with the elderly, carried out at least twice a week, promoted positive effects on the gain in flexion ROM of the hips and dorsiflexors as from four weeks of training.

The American College of Sport Medicine present recommendations for the prescription of stretching exercises, but they emphasize that the level of scientific evidence is still low (B and C), that is, it is based on studies carried out without a control group, without sample randomization and/or with a small number of participants, as described in Table 6.

This emphasizes the importance of flexibility training, considering that the majority of stretching techniques do not require specific localities or materials to carry them out, and are easy to understand (Gallo et al., 2012). In addition, studies reported in the literature have shown that the effects of stretching exercise can act as an important ally in the maintenance of the functional independence of the elderly (Batista et al., 2009; Cristopoliski et al., 2009; Stanziano et al., 2009; Watt et al., 2011; Zotz et al., 2014) such as: Gain in joint movement amplitude, gains in mobility and functionality, improvement in walking speed. Thus the implementation of flexibility training and the inclusion of stretching exercises in physical activity programs aimed at the elderly population, should be encouraged.

Prior to prescribing exercise, an individual evaluation of the older adult should be carried out to identify the objectives and the need and feasibility of carrying out stretching exercises, so that the prescription can be based on scientific evidence.

Table 5. Summary of the ACSM recommendations for flexibility exercises for older adults

Outcomes	Level of evidence
Duration of stretching for the older adults: 30-60s each repetition.	(C)
To increase movement amplitude, a total time of 60s for each grouping stretched.	(B)
2-3x/ week is sufficient to increase the ROM or flexibility.	(B)
Expressive gains are obtained with a daily stretching frequency.	(B)

(B) - Randomized controlled trials (limited body of data): Evidence is from end points of intervention studies that include only a limited number of randomized controlled trials (RCT), post hoc or subgroup analysis of RCT, or meta-analysis of RCT. In general, Category B pertains when few randomized trials exist, they are small in size, and the trial results are somewhat inconsistent, or the trials were undertaken in a population that differs from the target population of the recommendation; (C) - Nonrandomized trials, observational studies: Evidence is from outcomes of uncontrolled or nonrandomized trials or from observational studies (Chodzko-Zajko et al., 2009; Garber et al., 2011).

4. Balance and Sensoriomotor Training to Prevent Falls in the Elderly

4.1. Changes in Proprioception due to Ageing

Proprioception is a sensory modality involving the sense of body position in space and joint movement (Gandevia et al., 2002; Goble et al., 2009). It can also be defined as the capacity to perceive in a conscious or unconscious way, the movement and positioning of the joints by way of joint mechanoreceptors (Bacarin et al., 2004).

The term proprioception was introduced by Sherrington in 1906 to describe all neural information originating in the proprioceptors of the joints, muscles, tendons, capsules and ligaments, which are sent by way of the right-hand afferent innervation. The latter informs the central nervous system in a conscious or unconscious way, about the biomechanical relationships of the joint tissues which can influence muscle tone, motor and coordination execution programs, kinesthetics, muscle reflexes, postural balance and joint stability (Bacarin et al., 2004).

Sensory information derived from the visual, vestibular and somatosensory systems establish the postural control base, and a dysfunction in any part of these systems results in prejudice to postural control (Borin et al., 2010; Rogers, 2010). Proprioception is extremely important in the geriatric population, since deficits increase the risk of falls (Bacarin et al., 2004).

Due to biological ageing of the nervous system, the elderly present a reduced number of cutaneous and joint mechanoreceptors, which contributes to a reduction in the sense of joint position (Maki et al., 1999; Goble et al., 2009). The visual feedback can be compromised due to visual age-related diseases (cataract, glaucoma etc.) and in addition, the vestibular system is affected in about 30% of people over 70 (Impe et al., 2011; Rogers, 2010). All these factors contribute to a decrease in postural balance and can predispose the individual to falls.

In addition, senescence implies in peripheral changes such as demyelination, which appears to affect the sensory nerves first: A reduction in the sensitivity of the muscle spindle, alterations in the composition of the muscle spindle, including a reduction in fast myosin heavy chain isoforms and skin receptors (Goble, 2009).

In addition to these peripheral changes, the age-related decline in grey and white matter compromises the efficient integration of the different sensory inputs in the brain (Goble et al., 2009; Impe et al., 2011). Thus the decline in proprioception involves changes in both the central and peripheral nervous systems (Goble et al., 2009; Globe et al., 2012).

Goble et al., (2011) verified an increase in neural activity in the proprioception of the ankle in the elderly, for specific tasks in areas of the right-hand parietal lobe, frontal lobe, insular cortex and basal ganglion structures. These results confirm that, in addition to peripheral reflex mechanisms, the central processing of proprioceptive signs from the feet is fundamental for balance control. Thus such mapping could serve as balance control "biomarkers" in individuals with a balance deficit (Globe et al., 2011).

According to Suetterlin & Sayer (2014), the elderly show greater cortical activation than younger adults for the same tasks, and their proprioceptive acuity is more affected when their attention is divided, for example, in the case of a double task.

The decrease in proprioception with increase in age is a central factor for various geriatric syndromes, especially for falls, but it is relatively little considered in clinical practice (Lord, 1991). Thus a more precise clinical evaluation of proprioception is vital. Suetterlin & Sayer (2014) suggested the thumb finding and finger- nose tests, since they are easy to apply in a clinic, and also verification of the proprioceptive "biomarker" using functional magnetic nuclear resonance.

Apart from this, the evaluation of proprioceptive posture stability components could aid in the early detection of a decrease in anti-gravitational movements many years before the risk of falls becomes evident, so that an adequate proprioceptive control could be carried out and thus attenuate the effects of all the other fall risks (Riva et al., 2013).

A sedentary lifestyle accelerates the loss of proprioceptive acuity and thus contributes to a loss in functional independence and increase in falls in the elderly (Suetterlin, Sayer, 2014).

Thus public health strategies should aim at identifying elderly adults with non-modifiable risk factors for falls, such as feminine sex, since elderly women present a significantly greater decrease in balance than elderly men (Wu et al., 2013; Riva et al., 2013). Another strategy is to promote interventions to avoid the modifiable risk factors, such as: Low weight, central obesity with counselling on the control of sugar consumption by way of nutritional intervention, physical frailty by an adequate prescription of physical exercises, and a reduction in unnecessary medical prescriptions (Wu et al., 2013).

4.2. Prescription of Sensory-motor Exercises

Proprioception decreases with age, but physical exercise attenuates this loss (Ribeiro, Oliveira, 2007; Petrella, 2012). However, the exact mechanism which explains the improvement in proprioception promoted by exercise is still unknown, but it probably involves central and peripheral adaptations of the nervous system (Goble et al., 2009, Goble et al., 2012).

Table 6. Summary of recent studies analyzing the chronic effects of stretching in the aged (2009-2014)

Authors (year)	Sample	Training method	Volume/ duration of training	Joints trained	Evaluations	Results of training (just the variables that improved)
Cristopoliski et al., (2009)	20 elderly members of the community	Static passive	3x/week 4 repetitions Duration of each repetition: 60s 4 weeks (12 sessions)	Hip Ankle	Flexibility (photogrammetry)	Hip extension; uniarticular & biarticular hip flexion and ankle plantar flexion
Stanziano et al., (2009)	17 institutionalized elderly adults	FNP	2x/week 10 repetitions Duration of each repetition: 4-5s 8 weeks (16 sessions)	Shoulder Trunk Hip Ankle	Flexibility (chair-sit-and-reach & back-scratch test) Muscle strength of upper & lower limbs Agility Walking	Flexibility of upper & lower limbs; trunk rotation; knee extension; strength resistance of upper & lower limbs; strength power of lower limbs; agility & cardiorespiratory capacity
Gallon et al., (2011)	19 institutionalized elderly adults	Static active	3x/week 4 repetitions Duration of each repetition: 60s 8 weeks (24 sessions)	Hip	Flexibility & length of tendinous muscle (photogrammetry) Muscle strength (isokinetic dynamometer)	Uniarticular & biarticular hip flexion

Table 6. (Continued)

Authors (year)	Sample	Training method	Volume/ duration of training	Joints trained	Evaluations	Results of training (just the variables that improved)
Watt et al., (2011a)	82 elderly members of the community	Static passive	5x/week 4 repetitions Duration each repetition: 60s 10 weeks (50 sessions)	Hip	Flexibility (hip) Length of tendinous muscle Dynamic peak of hip extension Step length Walking speed	Walking speed, Dynamic peak of hip extension
Watt et al., (2011b)	74 fragile elderly adults	Static passive	5x/week 4 repetitions Duration each repetition: 60s 10 weeks (50 sessions)	Hip	Flexibility (hip) Length of tendinous muscle Dynamic peak of hip extension Step length Walking speed	Walking speed, Dynamic peak of hip extension
Gallo et al., (2013)	43 elderly members of the community	Static active	3x/week 3 repetitions: GT30 - 30s (each repetition) GT60 - 60s (each repetition) 16 weeks (48 sessions)	Shoulder Trunk Hip Ankle	Flexibility Coordination Agility Dynamic balance Resistance of muscle strength Aerobic resistance	Improvement in flexibility. Resistance of muscle strength, Aerobic resistance General index of functional aptitude.

Authors (year)	Sample	Training method	Volume/ duration of training	Joints trained	Evaluations	Results of training (just the variables that improved)
Bird et al., (2009)	32 elderly individuals	Resistance training (RT) Flexibility training (FT)	3x/ week (each training) RT: 3 series 10-12 repetitions (14-17 Borg) 4 weeks of wash out FT: 2 series, 20s 16 weeks each (40 sessions) Re-evaluated after 12 months	Ankle Knee Trunk	Muscle strength Static balance Flexibility	Improvements in muscle strength, balance and mobility were better in the group that continued the practice of resistance exercises.
Costa et al., (2013)	45 elderly individuals	Static active	2x/week 12 weeks (24 sessions in all) GA: 4 repetitions of 60s (each repetition) GR: 65% of 10RM GA + GR Re-evaluated after 6 weeks	Hip Ankle	ROM	Resistance exercises or stretching, carried out alone, are sufficient to increase ROM. Stretching was determinant for early gains and later maintenance after de-training

Table 6. (Continued)

Authors (year)	Sample	Training method	Volume/ duration of training	Joints trained	Evaluations	Results of training (just the variables that improved)
Locks et al., (2012)	45 elderly individuals	Static active	2x/week 12 weeks (24 sessions in all) GA: 4 repetitions of 60s (each repetition) GR: 65% of 10RM GA + GR Re-evaluated after 6 weeks	Hip	• Cardiorespiratory capacity • Muscle strength	6 weeks of resistance exercises or stretching improved functional performance. Systolic blood pressure reduced after 6 weeks of RE + stretching De-training (6 weeks) increased systolic BP when RE carried out alone.

Table 7. Summary of studies that verified the effect of virtual training in the elderly

Author, years	Design	Subjects	Intervention Group	Control Group	Variables evaluated	Conclusions
Bateni, 2012	CT Quasi experimental	n = 16	WG, n = 5	PG, n = 6, PWG, n = 5	BBS Bubble Test	PG and PWG had a great benefit on balance compared to WG.
Chen et al., 2012	Prospective, case controlled Non Randomized	n = 40	IG, n = 20	CG, n = 20	MFES, POMA; FRT; FTSS; TUG; Normalized MP; Normalized MVGRF; Maximum velocity; Total time; PP; RP; SP	The training reduced movement time, improved peak muscle power and balance.
Daniel, 2012	RCT	n = 19	WG, n = 7 SEG, n = 7	CG, n = 5	Rikli & Jones Tests; CHAMPS Physical Activity questionnaire; ABC Scale; LLFDI	The rehabilitation effects were similar for all groups.
Duque et al., 2013	RCT	n = 58	IG, n = 28	CG, n = 30	Postural Assessment (LOS, COP); Gait evaluation; Grip Strength; serum measurements; GDS; SAFFE; Mini-Nutritional Assessment	The BRU training is an effective method to complement other falls prevention and intervention programs in community-dwelling older fallers.

Table 7. (Continued)

Author, years	Design	Subjects	Intervention Group	Control Group	Variables evaluated	Conclusions
Franco et al., 2012	RCT	n = 31	WG, n = 11 MBG, n = 11	CG, n = 10	BBS, Tinetti Gait and Balance Assessment, SF-36; *Wii Fit* Enjoyment Questionnaire;	The interventions produced small improvements in balance. The duration of interventions was too short.
Laver et al., 2012	RCT	n = 44	WG, n = 22	PG, n = 22	TUG; SPPB; Modified BBS; Activities of Daily Living; Functional Independence Measure; ABC Scale; Quality of Life;	*Wii Fit* by physiotherapists with hospitalized older people is feasible with a small proportion of patients.
Lee et al., 2012	RCT	n = 55	IG, n = 27	CG,n = 28	Postural sway path length (anterior-posterior, medial-lateral and total measure) with eyes open and eyes closed.	VR exercise programs are suitable and effective preventing falls by elderly persons with type 2 diabetes.
Maillot et al., 2012	RCT	n = 30	IG, n = 15	CG, n = 15	BP; HR; Perceived exertion using the Borg scale; Rikli & Jones Tests; Cognitive battery.	Exergame training is an attractive activity and an effective way to promote physical and cognitive improvements among older adults.

Author, years	Design	Subjects	Intervention Group	Control Group	Variables evaluated	Conclusions
Pichierri et al., 2012a	RCT	n = 22	DG, n = 11	CG, n = 11	Foot placement accuracy, gait performance under single and dual task conditions.	Cognitive-motor intervention resulted in more improved gait under dual task conditions in comparison to a traditional strength and balance exercise program.
Pichierri et al., 2012b	RCT	n = 15	DG, n = 9	CG, n = 6	Voluntary step execution test.	Strength and balance exercises with additional dance video gaming improve voluntary step execution under single and dual task conditions.
Pluchino et al., 2012	RCT,	n = 27	WG, n = 8	BG, n = 11 TG, n = 8	TUG; One-Leg Stance; FRT; POMA; COP and time to boundary; DP; Falls Risk for Older People-community Setting and FES	VG was as effective as Tai Chi and the standard balance exercise program in improving postural control and balance.
Rendon et al., 2012	RCT	n = 40	IG, n = 20	CG, n = 20	8ft UG; ABC scale; GDS	*Wii Fit* gaming system improves balance and postural stability.
Singh et al., 2012	RCT	n = 36	WG, n = 18	BG, n = 18	PPA; ABC Scale.	VR exercise increase balance confidence and decrease risk of falls among community dwelling women.
Singh et al., 2013	RCT	n = 36	WG:18	BG:18	TST, OPI and TUG	VG training improves agility, balance and functional mobility.

Table 7. (Continued)

Author, years	Design	Subjects	Intervention Group	Control Group	Variables evaluated	Conclusions
Szturm et al., 2011	RCT	n = 27	IG, n = 14	BG, n = 13	BBS; TUG; ABC Scale; modified Clinical Test of Sensory Interaction and Balance; Spatial-temporal gait parameters.	VG improved dynamic standing balance control but there was no effect on gait function.
Toulotte et al., 2012	RCT	n = 36;	WG, n = 9 PAWG, n = 9	PAG, n = 9 CG, n = 9	Tinetti test, unipedal tests and the *Wii Fit*® tests	All training programs improved balance.

Characteristics of the studies involved in this review. - RCT: randomized controlled trial; CT: controlled trial; IG: intervention group; CG: control group; PG: physical therapy group; PWG: physical therapy and *Wii* group; DG: dance group; ABC Scale: activities-specific balance confidence scale; DSST: digit symbol substitution test; BP: blood pressure; HR: heart rate; BG: balance conventional group; TG: Tai Chi group; WG: *Wii* group; min: minutes; LLPR: human-computer interactive video-game based rehabilitation device; STS: speed sit-to-stand; MFES: modified falls efficacy scale; FRT: function reach test; FTSS: five times sit to stand; TUG: timed up and go; POMA: Tinetti Performance, Mobility Assessment; FES: Falls Efficacy Scale; COP: force plate center of pressure; DP: dynamic posturography; GDS: geriatric depression scale; 8ft UG: 8-foot up and go; MVGRF: maximal vertical ground reaction force; MP: maximum power; PP: preparation phase; RP: rising phase; SP: stabilization phase; SEG: seated exercise group; CHAMPS: community healthy activities model program for seniors; LLFDI: late life function and disability index; LOS: limits of stability; SAFFE: survey of activities and fear of falling in the elderly; BRU: Balance Rehabilitation Unit; VR: virtual reality; MBG: matter of balance group; SF-36: health survey short form; VO2: Maximum oxygen volume; SG: standard exercise group; SWG: standard exercise plus *Wii* group; NHPPT: the nursing home physical performance test; PACES: the original physical activity enjoyment scale; AROM: active range of motion; GPRC: global perceived rating of change; SPPB: short physical performance battery; PPA: physiological profile approach; PAG: physical activity group; PAWG: physical activity plus *Wii* group; TST: ten step test; OPI: overall performance index; VG: Video game. (Adapted from Rodrigues et al., 2014).

There is no evidence that exercise causes an increase in mechanoreceptors, but there are indications that training stimulates morphological adaptations in the main mechanoreceptor involving proprioception, the muscle spindle, such as metabolic changes in the intrafusal fibers, decrease in the latency of the stretch reflex and an increase in its amplitude (Goble et al., 2009).

According to Leporace et al., (2009), one should focus on the following four elements to reestablish sensory-motor deficits: Proprioception, dynamics stabilization, reactive neuromuscular control and functional motor patterns.

The mechanisms of proprioception involve both conscious and unconscious pathways. Thus the exercises prescribed should contain both conscious stimuli to stimulate cognition, and also sudden, unexpected changes in joint position to stimulate reflex muscle activity (Leporace et al., 2009). The prescribed exercises should involve balance on unstable surfaces while the individual is carrying out functional activities (Chodzko-Zajko et al., 2009; Leporace et al., 2009; Domingues et al., 2008; Page, 2006; Bandy, Sanders, 2003).

On the other hand, training in dynamic stabilization aims to improve the co-activation between antagonistic muscles. The exercises used to stimulate proprioception and dynamic stabilization should be carried out in a closed chain with small movements, since compression stimulates the joint receptors, and changes in the length-tension curve stimulate the muscle receptors (Leporace et al., 2009).

Limb repositioning exercises should also be carried out to stimulate the sense of joint position and neuromuscular control (Leporace et al., 2009).

1. Make the training postures progressively more difficult, so as to reduce the base support (example: 2-leg stance; semi-tandem; tandem; single leg stance)
2. Dynamic movements that upset the center of gravity (example: Walking in tandem; going round curves)
3. Make demands on postural muscles (Example: Remain on tip-toe)
4. Reduce the sensory input (Example: On foot with closed eyes)
5. Carry out sudden, unexpected changes in joint position
6. Exercises on unstable surfaces
7. Activity progression should be individualized and adapted according to tolerance and preference

Figure 3. Recommendations for the prescription of sensory-motor exercises for the elderly.

Reactive neuromuscular control is reached by way of exercises that create unexpected situations, such as perturbations on unstable surfaces when standing on one foot and when walking (Chodzko-Zajko et al., 2009; Leporace et al., 2009; Domingues et al., 2008; Page, 2006; Bandy, Sanders, 2003). Rhythmic stabilization exercises by way of the concept of Proprioceptive Neuromuscular Facilitation can also be used to improve reactive musculature control in addition to improving joint stability (Leporace et al., 2009).

Progression in sensory-motor training can be effected as from alterations in the exercise patterns carried out, starting with a 2-leg stance and progressing to a single leg stance, exercises with open eyes progressing to shut eyes and stimuli created by different surfaces (Chodzko-Zajko et al., 2009; Leporace et al., 2009; Domingues et al., 2008; Page, 2006; Bandy, Sanders, 2003).

According to the American College of Sports Medicine, Yoga and Tai Chi promote improvements in balance, agility, motor control, proprioception and quality of life in adults. However there are still no recommendations for neuromotor training due to the lack of studies, principally to determine the frequency, duration and intensity of the training programs. Some studies have suggested a frequency of two to three times a week with a duration of 20 to 30 minutes (Chodzko-Zajko et al., 2009).

For the elderly who are out of condition, functionally limited or suffering from chronic diseases that affect their capacity to carry out physical tasks, the intensity and duration of the physical activity should be limited. The progression of the activities should be individual and adapted to the individual's tolerance and preference, adopting a conservative approach. The muscle strengthening and/or balance training activities should precede the aerobic training activities amongst very frail individuals, and older adults should exceed the recommended minimum amounts of physical activity if they desire to improve their fitness. If the chronic conditions prevent carrying out the minimum amount of activity recommended, the individuals should carry out tolerated physical activities so as to avoid sedentarism (Garber et al., 2011).

Interventions including posture training and Tai Chi have shown a relationship with increased proprioceptive acuity in active seniors. However, in the future one should think about combining proprioceptive exercises with activities that generate increased cognitive demand in older adults, because this association enhances proprioceptive learning (Suetterlin, Sayer, 2014).

Rossi et al., (2013) showed that perturbation-based balance training, carried out three times a week for 6 weeks, improved the neuromuscular responses, such as ankle muscle reaction time and muscle activation, and consequently aided body capacity to maintain the correct pressure center. However, after a 6-week period of non-training, the gains were not maintained. Thus it can be seen that a lack of training can generate significant reductions in muscle reactive capacity and postural control, indicating that a progressive loss in postural and muscular capacity can occur in a relatively short period of time in elderly adults. This highlights the need for the aged to take part in regular exercise program (that is, without long pauses), so as to sustain the benefits obtained after the conclusion of an initial balance training program.

Another sensory motor training modality that has recently come into use is that of exercises carried out by way of a virtual interface. Nintendo® launched *Wii Fit* which consists of software based on exercises carried out by way of games, the console *Wii* and a specially developed controller the *Wii Balance Board* (WBB).

According to Nintendo, the objective of developing *Wii Fit* was to combine diversion with aptitude for all ages, including aspects of physical wellbeing such as joint flexibility, muscle strength and posture in the vertical position. The system is relatively cheap (~ US$200), easily accessible and the games are highly involving (Goble, Cone, Fling, 2014).

Various studies (Bateni, 2012; Chen et al., 2012; Daniel, 2012; Duque et al., 2013; Franco et al., 2012; Laver et al., 2012; Lee et al., 2012; Maillot et al., 2012; Pichierri et al., 2012a; Pichierri et al., 2012b; Pluchino et al., 2012; Rendon et al., 2012; Singh et al., 2012a; Singh et al., 2012b; Szturm et al., 2011; Toulotte et al., 2012) have shown improvements in static and dynamic balance, functional mobility, balance sway, walking and reaction time, and also in cognitive factors, using physical training by way of virtual games. However, differences in the exercise prescription parameters (such as training frequency, intensity and duration) with the use of video games in the studies, and also in the methods of evaluating the outcomes, limited the analysis of these studies (Table 7) (Rodrigues et al., 2014).

In addition one should emphasize the carrying out of controlled, randomized studies with an adequate sample size to investigate the neural and musculoskeletal adaptations resulting from the exercises carried out with virtual games, and make a comparison with other, commonly used balance interventions (Goble, Fing, 2014).

Considering the increasing evidence that proprioceptive acuity can be improved by way of training-based interventions, it is still a great challenge to determine which peripheral and/or central factors are associated with the age-related proprioceptive deficits. This will probably demand a combination of well- established protocols using the most advanced techniques such as neural recording and brain imaging, which could finally contribute to the development of more efficient strategies to improve the sensory-motor abilities of the elderly (Globe et al., 2009).

4.3. Prescription of Exercises for Hip and Knee Osteoarthritis

Single leg stance exercises can be used to increase hip bone density, improve postural balance and prevent falls in the elderly. These outcomes were observed in a protocol that emphasized support for one minute on each lower limb with the eyes open, holding on to a support or otherwise, carried out 3 times a day (morning, afternoon and night) for 3 months (Sakamoto et al., 2006).

In a protocol carried out once a day with progressive resistance strength training, with prior warming up constituted of 5 repetitions of knee extension with no load, 3 series of 10 repetitions with 1 minute of rest between each series, the intensity (weight/load) evaluated using the 10 repetition maximum (10RM) test in each session for knee extenders, starting between the 2nd and 4th days after total arthroplasty of the hip surgery in the elderly, showed a decrease in the difference in strength between the operated limb and the healthy contralateral limb, without interfering with the painful scenario (Kronborg et al., 2014).

In a systematic review of the guidelines for recommendations for the treatment of knee OA, the reviewers found strong evidence for the use of strength, aerobic and balance (tai chi & yoga) exercises and combined exercises (Larmer et al., 2014). Laser therapy, magnetic bracelets, Chinese acupuncture, therapeutic massage, psychosocial therapy and electro-acupuncture were not recommended, considering the studies cited in this review (Larmer et al., 2014).

It was verified that exercise programs for the treatment of knee OA should concentrate on improving aerobic capacity, quadriceps muscle strength or the performance of the lower limbs. For patients with low muscle strength aerobic capacity, aerobic exercises and strength training should be carried out on different days in order to attain the best effect. For better results the program should be supervised, carried out three times a week and include at least 12 sessions. The exercise program should be carried out independent of the patient's characteristics, including the radiographic severity and initial pain (Juhl et al., 2014).

In another systematic review with a meta-analysis, it was shown that strength treatment, principally of the knee extensors, Tai Chi and aerobic exercises improved the balance and risk of falling in elderly patients with knee OA, whereas exercises carried out in the water and mild treatments did not significantly improve the balance results (Mat et al., 2014).

Thus it was shown that strength treatment, Tai Chi and aerobic exercises could be recommended as strategies to prevent falls and for the treatment of individuals with knee OA.

For the post-operative treatment of total knee arthroplasty (TKA), protocols of progressive exercises and the early (2 days after the operation) application of neuromuscular electrical stimulation (NMES) should be carried out to attenuate weakness of the quadriceps and associated problems. The rehabilitation protocol should include: Progressive strength exercises for the quadriceps and intensive functional exercises carried out on the ground or in an aquatic medium. The treatment should be individualized and supervised by a physiotherapist in order to obtain the best treatment after TKA on a short or long term basis. The exercise program should last for a minimum of 12 supervised sessions of strength training, but further studies are required to define: Dose, frequency, intensity and criteria for progression (Pozzy, Snyder-Mackler, Zeni, 2013).

Hip TA:
• Progressive resistance strengthening exercise for knee extensors; • Start 2 to 4 days after surgery; • Once a day; • Warming up: 5 repetitions of knee extension with no load; • Prescription: 3 series of 10 repetitions with 1minute of rest between each series, the intensity (weight/load) being evaluated by the 10RM test in each session.
Knee TA:
• Prior application (2 days post-operative) of NMES; • Quadriceps strengthening exercises, progressive according to patient improvement; • Sensory-motor exercises: 12 x 60 minute sessions using exercises with balance perturbation (side walking, cross walking, walking with change in direction, foam activities, tilt board activities, roller board and platform perturbations); 15 minutes of *Wii Fit*® training associated with 60 minutes of conventional physiotherapy.

Figure 4. Summary of the exercises for Total Arthroplasy (TA) of the hip and knee.

Hip OA: ✓ There is no evidence for the treatment of hip OA, but it is believed that supervised therapeutic exercises based on strength training are indicated for its treatment.
Knee OA: ❖ Strength training principally for the knee extensors; ❖ Tai Chi; ❖ Aerobic exercises; ❖ Supervised exercises, 3 times a week; ❖ 12 sessions.

Figure 5. Summary of the prescription of exercises for hip & knee OA.

In addition to the decrease in strength of the quadriceps, individuals submitted to TKA show a great loss of balance, which increases the risks of falls and new injuries. Thus after TKA, sensory-motor exercises should be considered in the prescription of exercises for post-operative TKA (Pozzy, Snyder-Mackler, Zeni, 2013).

The authors point out that balance exercises with perturbation carried out for at least 12 sixty-minute sessions, promote an improvement in the functional parameters verified in the following tests: Forward reach, single leg stance, sit-to-stand test, stair climbing time, 10m walk time and TUG scores. The exercises that use interactive technologies such as *Wii Fit*® are also indicated for the post-surgery treatment of TKA for at least 15 minutes, associated with conventional physiotherapy (Pozzy, Snyder-Mackler, Zeni, 2013).

With respect to hip OA, more research is required to confirm if the exercises are beneficial to the hip muscles and to the population with hip OA (Zacharias et al., 2014). However, therapeutic and supervised exercise training with an element of strengthening is an efficacious treatment for hip OA (Bennell & Hinman, 2011).

Since the prevalence of OA should double by 2020 and the personal and social costs associated with OA will be substantial, it is important to establish the best strategy to control and treat it. Physical exercise plus orientations show strong evidence of doing just this at relatively low cost, and thus this is an opportunity for professionals involved with rehabilitation to lead the management of OA (Larmer et al., 2014).

Conclusion

Although the ageing process is accompanied by a series of alterations in musculoskeletal structure and function, which frequently predispose the aged to diseases such as sarcopenia and osteoarthritis, the regular practice of physical exercise appears as the main non-pharmacological intervention for the prevention of such diseases and the improvement in functional outcomes such as muscle strength, balance and a reduction in the risk of falls, providing an improvement in the quality of life of elderly adults.

References

Ali, S., Garcia, J. M. Sarcopenia, Cachexia and Aging: Diagnosis, mechanisms and therapeutic options: A mini-review. *Gerontol.* 2014; 60: 294-305.

Bacarin, T. A., Sacco, I. C. N., Kageyama, E. R. R. O., Yogi, L. S. Propriocepção na artroplastia total de joelho em idosos: Uma revisão de literatura. *Rev Fisioter Univ São Paulo,* 2004; 11(2): 96-104.

Ballak, S. B., Degens, H., de Haan, A., Jaspers, R. T. Ageing related changes in determinants of muscle force generating capacity: A comparison of muscle aging in men and male rodents. *Ageing Res Rev.* 2014; 14:43-55.

Bandy, W. D., & Sanders, B. *Exercício Terapêutico Técnicas para intervenção.* Guanabara Koogan: Rio de Janeiro, 2003.

Baranda, P. S., Ayala, F. Chronic flexibility improvement after 12 week of stretching program utilizing the ACSM recommendations: Hamstring Flexibility. *International Journal of Sports Medicine,* 2010; 31(6):389-96.

Baroni, B. M., Geremia, J. M., Rodrigues, R. et al., Functional and morphological adaptations to aging in knee extensor muscles of physically active men. *Journal of applied biomechanics.* 2013; 29(5):535-42.

Bateni, H. Changes in balance in older adults based on use of physical therapy vs. the *Wii Fit* gaming system: A preliminary study. *Physiotherapy.* 2012; 98(3): 211-6.

Batista, L. H., Vilar, A. C., de Almeida Ferreira, J. J., Rebelatto, J. R., Salvini, T. F. Active stretching improves flexibility, joint torque, and functional mobility in older women. *Am J Phys Med Rehabil,* 2009;88(10):815-22.

Bennell K. L., Hinman R. S. A review of the clinical evidence for exercise in osteoarthritis of the hip and knee. *J Sci Med Sport.* 2011; 14(1):4-9.

Bergman, H., Béland, F., Karunananthan, S., Hummel, S., Hogan, D., Wolfson, C. Canadian iniciative on frailty and aging. Developing a working framework for understanding frailty. *Gerontol Soc.* 2004; 109:15-29.

Bird, M. L., Hill, K., Ball, M., Williams, A. D. Effects of resistance- and flexibility-exercise interventions on balance and related measures in older adults. *J Aging Phys Act,* 2009;17(4):444-54.

Boakes J. L., Foran J., Ward S. R., Lieber R. L. Muscle adaptation by serial sarcomere addition 1 year after femoral lengthening. *Clin Orthop Relat Res.* 2007; (456):250-3.

Borin, G., Masullo, C. L., Bonfim, T. R. et al., Controle postural em pacientes com lesão do ligamento cruzado anterior. *Fisioter Pesqui.* 2010; 17(4): 342-5.

Boyer, K. A., Andriacchi, T. P., Beaupre, G. S. The role of physical activity in changes in walking mechanics with age. *Gait Posture.* 2012; 36(1):149-53.

Callisaya, M. L., Blizzard, L., Schmidt, M. D., Mcginley, J. L., Lord, S. R., Srikanth, V. K. A population-based study of sensoriomotor factors affecting gait in older people. *Age Ageing,* 2009; 38:290-295.

Carroll, C. C., Dickinson, J. M., Haus, J. M., et al., Influence of aging on the *in vivo* properties of human patellar tendon. *Journal of Applied Physiology,* 2008; 105: 1907-1915.

Chen, H. C., Schultz, A. B., Ashton-Miller, J. A., Giordani, B., Alexander, N. B., Guire, K. E. Stepping over obstacles: Dividing attention impairs performance of old more than young adults. *J Gerontol.* 1996; 5I (3) M116-22.

Chen, P. Y., Wei, S. H., Hsieh, W. L., Cheen, J. R., Chen, L. K., Kao, C. L. Lower limb power rehabilitation (LLPR) using interactive video game for improvement of balance function in older people. *Arch Gerontol Geriatr.* 2012; 55(3):677-82.

Clark, B., Manini, T. B. Sarcopenia ≠ Dynapenia. *J Gerontol.* 2008; 63(8):829-834.

Chodzko-Zajko, M. J. N. Proctor, D. N., Singh, M. A. F., Minson, C. T., Nigg, C. R., Salem, G. J., Skinner, J. S. Exercise and Physical Activity for Older Adults. *Med Sci Sports Exerc,* 2009; 1510-1530.

Christiansen, C. L. The effects of hip and ankle stretching on gait function of older people. *Arch Phys Med Rehabil,* 2008; 89 (8):1421-8.

Clemson, L., Mackenzie, L., Ballinger, C., Close, J. C. T., Cumming, R. G. Environmental interventions to prevent falls in community-dwelling older people: A meta-analysis of randomized trials. *Aging Health.* 2008; 20:954-971.

Cofré, L. E., Lythgo, N., Morgan, D., Galea, M. P. Aging modifies joint power and work when gait speeds are matched. *Gait Posture.* 2011 Mar; 33(3):484-9.

Cooper, R., Mishra, G., Clennell, S., Guralnik, J., Kuh, D. Menopausal status and physical performance in midlife: Findings from a British birth cohort study. *Menopause.* 2008; 15:1079-1085.

Costa, T. C., Locks, R. R., Koppe, S., Yamaguti, A. M., Formiga, A., Gomes, A. R. S. Strength And Stretching Training And Detraining On Flexibility Of Elderly. *Top Geriatr Rehabil.* 2013; 29:142-148.

Couppé, C., Hansen, P., Kongsgaard, M. et al., Mechanical properties and collagen cross-linking of the patellar tendon in old and young men. *Journal of Applied Physiology,* 2009;107: 880-886.

Coutinho, E. L., de Luca, C., Salvini, T. F., Vidal, B. C. Bouts of passive stretching after immobilization of the rat soleus muscle increase collagen macromolecular organization and muscle fiber area. *Connect Tissue Res.* 2006; 47(5):278-286.

Coutinho, E. L., Gomes, A. R. S., França, C. N., Oishi, J., Salvini, T. F. Effect of passive stretching on the immobilized soleus muscle fiber morphology. *Brazilian J Med Biol Res.* 2004; 37:1853-1861.

Cristopoliski, F., Barela, J. A., Leite, N., Fowler, N. E., Rodacki, A. L. et al., Stretching exercise program improves gait in the elderly. *Gerontol.* 2009; 55(6):614-20.

Cruz-Jentoft, A. J., Baeyens, J. P., Bauer, J. et al., M. Sarcopenia: European consensus on definition and diagnosis. *Age Ageing.* 2010; 39:412-423.

Daniel K. Wii-hab for pre-frail older adults. *Rehabil Nurs.* 2012; 37(4):195-201.

Dionne, I. J., Kinaman, K. A., Poehlman, E. T. Sarcopenia and muscle function during menopause and hormone-replacement therapy. *J Nutr Health Aging,* 2000; 4:156-161.

Dodson, S., Baracos, V. E., Jatoi, A., Evans, W. J., Cella, D., Dalton, J. T., Steiner, M. S. Muscle Wasting in Cancer Cachexia: Clinical Implications, Diagnosis, and Emerging Treatment Strategies. *Annu Rev Med.* 2011; 62: 265-279.

Delbaere, K., Sturnieks, D. L., Crombez, G., Lord, S. R. Concern about falls elicits changes in gait parameters in conditions of postural threat in older people. *J Gerontol A Biol Sci Med Sci.* 2009; 64(2):237-242.

De Vita, P., Hortobagyi, T. Age causes a redistribution of joint torques and powers during gait. *J Appl Physiol.* 2000; 88(5):1804-11.

Doherty, T. J. Physiology of aging. Invited review: Aging and sarcopenia. *J Appl Physiol.* 2003; 95: 1717-27.

Domingues, M. L. P. Treino Proprioceptivo na Prevenção e Reabilitação de Lesões nos Jovens Atletas. *Motriz.* 2008; 4(4):29-37.

Doriot, N., Wang, X. Effects of age and gender on maximum voluntary range of motion of the upper body joints. *Ergonomics.* 2006. 22; 49(3):269-81.

Duque, G., Boersma, D., Loza-Diaz, G., Hassan, S., Suarez, H., Geisinger, D. et al., Effects of balance training using a virtual-reality system in older fallers. *Clin Interv Aging.* 2013; 8:257-63.

Evans, W. J., Morley, J. E., Argiles, J., Bales, C., Baracos, V., Guttridge, D. et al., Cachexia: A new definition. *Clin Nutr.* 2008; 27:793-799.

Feland, J. B., Myrer, J. W., Schulthies, S. S., Fellingham, G. W., Measom, G. W. The effect of duration of stretching of the hamstring muscle group for increasing range of motion in people aged 65 years or older. *Phys Ther,* 2001; 81(5):1110-7.

Ferrucci, L., Guralnik, J., Studenski, S., Fried, L., Cutler, G., Walston, J. et al., Designing randomized, controlled trials aimed at preventing or delaying functional decline and disability in frail, older persons: A consensus report. *J Am Geriatr Soc.* 2004; 52:625-34.

Franco J. R., Jacobs K., Inzerillo C., Kluzik J. The effect of the Nintendo *Wii Fit* and exercise in improving balance and quality of life in community dwelling elders. *Technol Health Care.* 2012; 20(2):95-115.

Fried, L, P., Tangen, C. M., Walston, J. et al., Frailty in older adults: Evidence for a phenotype. *J Gerontol A Biol Sci Med Sci.* 2001; 56(3):146-56.

Fried, L. P., Walston, J. *Frailty and failure to thrive.* In: Hazzard, W. R., Blass, J. P., Ettinger, W. H., Halter, J. B., Ouslander. J. Principles of Geriatric Medicine and Gerontology. 4th ed. New York: McGraw Hill. 1998:1387–1402.

Frontera, W. R., Suh, D., Krivickas, L. S., Hughes, V. A., Goldstein, R., Roubenoff, R. Skeletal muscle fiber quality in older men and women. *J Physiol. Cell Physiology,* Bethesda, 2000; 279(3): C611-C618.

Frontera, W. R., Reid, K. F., Phillips, E. M., Krivickas, L. S., Hughes, V. A., Roubenoff, R., Fielding R. A. Muscle fiber size and function in elderly humans: A longitudinal study. *J Appl Physiol,* 2008; 105:637-642.

Fukumoto, Y., Ikezoe, T., Yamada, Y., Tsukagoshi, R., Nakamura, M., Mori, N., Kimura, M., Ichihashi, N. Skeletal muscle quality assessed from echo intensity is associated with muscle strength of middle-aged and elderly persons. *Eur J Appl Physiol.* 2012; 112(4):1519-25.

Gallo, L. H., Gobbi, S., Gonçalves, R., Jambassi Filho, J. C., Prado, A. K. G., Ceccato, M., Gurjão, A. L. D., Gobbi, L. T. B. Alongamento no Programa de Atividade Física para Terceira Idade (PROFIT): Promovendo a melhora da capacidade funcional em idosas. *Revista de Terapia Ocupacional da Universidade de São Paulo,* São Paulo, 2012; 23(1)1-6.

Gallo, L. H., Gonçalves, R., Gurjão, A. L. D., Prado, A. K. G., Ceccato, M. J., Jambassi Filho, C., Gobbi, S. Effect of different stretching volumes on functional capacity in elderly women. *Rev Bras Cineantropom Desempenho Hum.* 2013;15(1):103-112.

Gallon, D., Rodacki, A. L., Hernandez, S. G., Drabovski, B., Outi, T., Bittencourt, L. R. et al., The effects of stretching on the flexibility, muscle performance and functionality of institutionalized older women. *Braz J Med Biol Res.* 2011; 44(3):229-35.

Gajdosik, R. L., Vander Linden, D. W., Mcnair, P. J., Riggin, T. J., Albertson, J. S., Mattick, D. J. C. et al., Slow passive stretch and release characteristics of the calf muscles of older women with limited dorsiflexion range of motion. *Clin Biomech.* 2004; 19(4):398-406.

Gajdosik, R. L., Vander Linden, D. W., Mcnair, P. J., Williams, A. K., Riggin, T. J. Effects of an eight-week stretching program on the passive-elastic properties and function of the calf muscles of older women. *Clin Biomech.* 2005;20(9):973-83.

Garber, C. E., Blissmer, B., Deschenes, M. R., Franklin, B. A., Lamonte, M. J., Lee, I. M., Nieman, D. C., Swain, D. P. Quantity and Quality of Exercise for Developing and Maintaining Cardiorespiratory, Musculoskeletal, and Neuromotor Fitness in Apparently Healthy Adults: Guidance for Prescribing Exercise. *Med Sci Sports Exerc.* 2011; 43(7): 1334-1359.

Goble, D. J., Cone, B. L., Fling, B. W. Using the *Wii Fit* as a tool for balance assessment and neurorehabilitation: The first half decade of "*Wii*-search". *J Neuroeng Rehabil.* 2014,11:12.

Goble, D. J., Coxon, J. P., Wenderoth, N., van Impe, A., Swinnen, S. P. Proprioceptive sensibility in the elderly: Degeneration, functional consequences and plastic-adaptive processes. *Neurosc Biobehav Ver.* 2009; 33,271-278.

Goble, D. J., Coxon, J. P., van Impe, A., Geurts, M., Doumas, M., Wenderoth, N., Swinnen, S. P. Brain Activity during Ankle Proprioceptive Stimulation

Predicts Balance Performance in Young and Older Adults. *J Neurosci.* 2011; 31(45):16344-16352.

Goble, D. J., Coxon, J. P., van Impe, A., Geurts, M., van Hecke, W., Sunaert, S., Wenderoth, N., Swinnen, S. P. The Neural Basis of Central Proprioceptive Processing in Older Versus Younger Adults: An Important Sensory Role for Right Putamen. *Hum Brain Mapp.* 2012; 33: 895-908.

Guimarães, J. M. N., Farinatti, P. T. V. Análise descritiva de variáveis teoricamente associadas ao risco de quedas em mulheres idosas. *Rev Bras Med Esporte.* 2005; 11(5):299-305.

Hall, D. T., Ma, J. F., Marco, S. D., Gallouzi, I. E. Inducible nitric oxide synthase (iNOS) in muscle wasting syndrome, sarcopenia and cachexia. *Aging.* 2011; 3(8):1-14.

Hasson, C. J., van Emmerik R. E. A., Caldwell, G. E. Balance Decrements are Associated With Age-Related Muscle Property Changes. *J Appl Biomech.* 2014; 30(4):555-62.

Horak, F. B. Postural orientation and equilibrium: What do we need to know about neural control of balance to prevent falls? *Age Ageing.* 2006; 35 Suppl 2:ii7-ii11.

Izquierdo, M., Ibañez, J., Gorostiaga, E., Garrues, M., Zúñiga, A., Antón, A., Larrión, J. L., Häkkinen, K. Maximal strength and power characteristics in isometric and dynamic actions of the upper and lower extremities in middle-aged and older men. *Acta Physiol Scand.* 1999 Sep; 167(1):57-68.

Juhl, C., Christensen, R., Roos, E. M., Zhang, W., Lund, H. Impact of Exercise Type and Dose on Pain and Disability in Knee Osteoarthritis: A Systematic Review and Meta-Regression Analysis of Randomized Controlled Trials. *Arthritis Rheumatol.* 2014; 66(3):622-636.

Kadi, F., Karlsson, C., Larsson, B., Eriksson, J., Larva, M., Billig, H., Jonsdottir, I. H. The effects of physical activity and estrogen treatment on rat fast and slow skeletal muscles following ovariectomy. *J Muscle Res Cell Motil,* 2002; 23:335-339.

Kamikawa, Y., Ikeda, S., Harada, K., Ohwatashi, A., Yoshida, A. Passive Repetitive stretching for a short duration within a week increases myogenic regulatory factors and myosin heavy chain mRNA in rats' skeletal muscle. *The Scientific World Journal,* 2013; 1-6.

Kerrigan, D. C., Xenopoulos-Oddsson, A., Sullivan, M. J., Lelas, J. J., Riley, P. O. Effect of a hip flexor-stretching program on gait in the elderly. *Arch Phys Med Rehabil.* 2003; 84(1):1-6.

Klaas, A., Hartholt, K. A., Polinder, S., van der Cammen, T. J. M., Panneman, M. J. M., van der Velde, N., van Lieshout, E. M. M., Patka, P., van Beeck,

E. F. Costs of falls in an ageing population: A nationwide study from the Netherlands (2007-2009). *Injury, Int. J. Care Injured.* 2012:43, 1199-1203.

Khalaj, N., Osman, N. A. A., Mokhtar, A. H., Mehdikhani, M., Wan Abas, W. A. B. Balance and Risk of Fall in Individuals with Bilateral Mild and Moderate Knee Osteoarthritis. *PLoS ONE* 9(3): e92270. doi: 10.1371/journal.pone.0092270.

König, N., Taylor, W. R., Armbrecht, G., Dietzel, R., Singh, N. B. Identification of functional parameters for the classification of older female fallers and prediction of 'first-time' fallers. *J. R. Soc. Interface.* 2014; 11: 20140353.

Konrad, A., Tilp, M. Increased range of motion after static stretching is not due to changes in muscle tendon structures. *Clin Biomech.* 2014.

Kokkonen, J., Nelson, A. G., Eldredge, C., Winchester, J. B. Chronic static stretching improves exercise performance. *Med Sci Sports Exerc.* 2007; 39(10):1825-31.

Kokkonen, J., Nelson, A. G., Cornwell, A. Acute muscle stretching inhibits maximal strength performance. *Res Q Exerc Sport.* 1998; 69(4):411-15.

Kragstrup, T. W., Kjaer, M., Mackey, A. L. Structural, Biochemical, cellular and functional changes in skeletal muscle extracellular matrix with aging. *Scand J Med Scienc Sports,* 2011; 21:749-757.

Kronborg, L., Bandholm, T., Palm, H., Kehlet, H., Kristensen, M. T. Feasibility of progressive strength training implemented in the acute ward after hip fracture surgery. *PLoS One.* 2014; 9(4):e93332.

Kulmala, J. P., Korhonen, M. T., Kuitunen, S., Suominen, H., Heinonen, A., Mikkola, A., Avela, J. Which muscles compromise human locomotor performance with age? *J R Soc Interface.* 2014; 6; 11(100):20140858.

Kumar, A., Carpenter, H., Morris, R., Iliffe, S., Kendrick, D. Which factors are associated with fear of falling in community-dwelling older people? *Age Ageing.* 2014; 43(1):76-84.

Larmer, P. J., Reay, N. D., Aubert, E. R., Kersten, P. Systematic Review of Guidelines for the Physical Management of Osteoarthritis. *Arch Phys Med Rehabil.* 2014; 95:375-89.

Laver K., George S., Ratcliffe J. et al., Use of an interactive video gaming program compared with conventional physiotherapy for hospitalized older adults: A feasibility trial. *Disabil Rehabil Assist Technol.* 2012; 34(21): 1802-1808.

Lee S. W., Song C. H., Virtual Reality Exercise Improves Balance of Elderly Persons with Type 2 Diabetes: A Randomized Controlled Trial *J. Phys. Ther. Sci.* 2012; 24:261-265.

Leonard, C. T., Matsumoto, T., Diedrich, P. M., Mcmillan, J. A. Changes in neural modulation and motor control during voluntary movement of older individuals. *J Gerontol.* 1997; 52(5).

Leporace, G., Metsavaht, L., Sposito, MMM. Importância do treinamento da propriocepção e do controle motor na reabilitação após lesões músculo-esqueléticas. *Acta Fisiatr.* 2009; 16(3):126-131.

Lieber, R. L., Fridén, J. Functional and clinical significance of skeletal muscle architecture. *Muscle Nerve.* 2000; 23(11):1647-66.

Lord, S. R., Clark, R. D., Webster, I. W. Postural stability and associated physiological factors in a population of aged persons. *J Gerontol.* 1991; 46(3):M69-76.

Lord, S. R., Lloyd, D. G., Li, S. K. Sensori-motor Function, Gait Patterns and Falls in Community-dwelling Women. *Age Ageing.* 1996; 25:292-299.

Lord, S. R., Murray, S. M., Chapman, K., Munro, B., Tiedemann, A. Sit-to-stand performance depends on sensation, speed,balance and psychological status in addition to strength inolder people. *J Gerontol,* 2002; 57:M539-43.

Macedo, C., Gazzola, J. M., Najas, M. Frailty syndrome in elderly patients: The importance of physiotherapy. *Arq. Bras. Cienc Saúde.* 2008; 33(3): 177-84.

Macedo, A. C. B., Ywazaki, J. L., Pacheco, J., Gonçalves, S., Goes, A. R. S. Acute effects of gastrocnemius muscle stretching after contusion in rats. *Fisioter Pesq.* 2014; 21(1):53-59.

Magnusson, S. P., Simonsen, E. B., Dyhre-Poulsen, P., Aagaard, P., Mohr, T., Kjaer, M. Viscoelastic stress relaxation during static stretch in human skeletal muscle in the absence of EMG activity. *Scand J Med Sci Sports,* 1996;6:323-8.

Maillot P., Perrot A., Hartley A. Effects of interactive physical-activity video-game training on physical and cognitive function in older adults. *Psychol Aging.* 2012; 27(3):589-600.

Maki, B. E., Perry, S. D., Norrie, R. G., Mcllroy, W. E. Effect of Facilitation of Sensation From Plantar Foot-Surface Boundaries on Postural Stabilization in Young and Older Adults. *J Gerontol.* 1999:54(6), 281-287.

Maltais M. L., Desroches J., Dionne I. J. Changes in muscle mass and strength after menopause. *J Musc Neur Interact,* 2009; 9:186-197.

Mat, S., Tan, M., Kamaruzzaman, S. B., Ng, C. T. Physical therapies for improving balance and reducing falls risk in osteoarthritis of the knee: A systematic review. *Age Ageing.* 2014; 0:1-9.

Mattielo-Sverzut A. C., Petersen S. G., Kjaer M., Mackey A. L. Morphological adaptation of muscle collagen and receptor of advances glycation end product (RAGE) in osteoarthritis patients with 12 weeks of resistance training: Influence of anti-inflammatory or glucosamine treatment. *Rheumatol Int.* 2013; 33:2215-2224.

Melzer, I., Benjuya, B., Kaplanski, J. Postural stability in the elderly: A comparison between fallers and non-fallers. *Age Ageing.* 2004; 33:602-607.

Miszko, T. A., Cress, M. E., Slade, J. M., Covey, C. J., Agrawal, S. K., Doerr, C. E. Effect of strength and power training on physical function in community-dwelling onder adults. *J Gerontol A Biol Med Sci,* 2003; 58(2):171-175.

Monaco, V., Rinaldi, L. A., Macrì, G., Micera, S. During walking elders increase efforts at proximal joints and keep low kinetics at the ankle. *Clin Biomech* (Bristol, Avon). 2009; 24(6):493-8.

Moretto, M. C., Alves, R. M. A., Neri, A. L., Guariento, M. E. Relationship between nutritional status and frailty in Brazilian elderly. *Rev Bras Clin Med.* 2012; 10(4):167-71.

Morse, C. I., Thom, J. M., Birch, K. M. et al., Changes in triceps surae muscle architecture with sarcopenia. *Acta Physiol Scand,* 2005; 183:291-8.

Muscaritoli, M., Anker, S. D., Argilés, J., Aversa, Z., Bauer, J. M. et al., Consensus definition of sarcopenia, cachexia and pre-cachexia: Joint document elaborated by Special Interest Groups (SIG) ''cachexia-anorexia in chronic wasting diseases'' and ''nutrition in geriatrics''. *Clin Nutri.* 2010; 29: 15-159.

Narici, M. V., Maganaris, C. N., Reeves, N. D., Capodaglio. Effect of aging on human architecture. *J Appl Physiol.* 2003; 95(6):2229- 2234.

Narici, M. V., Maganaris, C. N. Plasticity of the muscle-tendon complex with disuse and aging. *Exerc Sport Sci Rev.* 2007; 35(3):126-34.

Narici, M. V., Maffulli, N. Sarcopenia: Characteristics, mechanisms and functional significance. *Br Med Bull.* 2010:95:139-159.

Neri, A. L., Yassuda, M. S., Araújo, L. F., Eulálo, M. C., Cabral, B. E., Siqueira, M. E. C., Santos, G. A., Moura, J. G. A. Metodologia e perfil sociodemográfico, cognitivo e de fragilidade de idosos comunitários de sete cidades brasileiras: Estudo FIBRA. *Cad Saude Pub.* 2013; 29(4):778-779.

Page, P. Sensorimotor training: A ''global'' approach for balance training. *J Body Mov Ther.* 2006; 10: 77-84.

Palus, S., von Haeling, S., Springer, J. Muscle Wasting: An overview of recent developments in basic research. *J Cachexia Sarcop Muscle.* 2014; 5:193-198.

Petterson, S. C., Mizner, R. L., Stevens, J. E., Raisis, L., Bodenstab, A., Newcomb, W., Snyder-Mackler, A. Improved Function from Progressive Strengthening Interventions after Total Knee Arthroplasty: A Randomized Clinical Trial with an Imbedded Prospective Cohort. *Arthritis Care Research.* 2009:61(2):174-183.

Petrella, M., Neves, T. M., Reis, J. G., Gomes, M. M., Oliveira, R. D. R., Abreu, D. C. C. Parâmetros do controle postural em mulheres idosas com ou sem histórico de quedas associadas ou não à osteoartrite de joelhos. *Rev Bras Reumatol.* 2012a; 52(4):507-517.

Pichierri, G., Murer, K., de Bruin, E. D. A cognitive-motor intervention using a dance video game to enhance foot placement accuracy and gait under dual task conditions in older adults: A randomized controlled trial. *BMC Geriatr.* 2012a; 12(74):1471-2318.

Pichierri, G., Coppe, A., Lorenzetti, S., Murer, K., de Bruin, E. D. The effect of a cognitive-motor intervention on voluntary step execution under single and dual task conditions in older adults: A randomized controlled pilot study. *Clin Interv Aging.* 2012b; 7:175-84.

Pijnappels, M., van der Burg, P. J., Reeves, N. D., van Dieen, J. H. Identification of elderly fallers by muscle strength measures. *Eur J Appl Physiol.* 2008; 102(5):585-92.

Pluchino, A., Lee, S. Y., Asfour, S., Roos, B. A., Signorile, J. F. Pilot study comparing changes in postural control after training using a video game balance board program and 2 standard activity-based balance intervention programs. *Arch Phys Med Rehabil.* 2012; 93(7):1138-46.

Pozzi, F., Snyder-Mackler, L., Zeni J. Physical exercise after knee arthroplasty: A Systematic review of controlled trials. *Eur J Phys Rehabil Med.* 2013; 49(6):877-892.

Proske, U., Wise, A. K., Gregory, J. E. The role of muscle receptors in the detection of movements. *Prog Neurobiol.* 2000:60; 85-96.

Rendon A. A., Lohman E. B., Thorpe D., Johnson E. G., Medina E., Bradley B. The effect of virtual reality gaming on dynamic balance in older adults. *Age Ageing.* 2012; 41: 549-552.

Ribeiro, F., Oliveira J. Efeito da fadiga muscular local na propriocepção do joelho. *Fisioter. Mov.* 2008, 21(2):71-83.

Ribeiro, F., Oliveira J. Ageing effects on joint proprioception: The role of physical activitiy in proprioception conservation. *Eur Rev Aging Phys Act.* 2007; 4:71-76.

Riva, D., Mamo, C., Fanì, M., Saccavino, P., Rocca, F., Momenté, M., Fratta, M. Single Stance Stability and Proprioceptive Control in Older Adults Living at Home: Gender and Age Differences. *J Aging Res.* 2013, Article ID 561695.

Rocha, O. M., Batista, A. A. P., Maesta, N., Burini, R. C., Laurindo, I. M. M. Sarcopenia da caquexia reumatoide: Conceituação, mecanismos, consequências clinicas e tratamentos possíves. *Ver Bras Reumatol.* 2009; 49(3):288-301.

Rocha, N. P., Reis, H. J., Teixeira, A. L. *Inflammaging:* Um novo paradigma para as ciências gerontológicas. *Geriatr Gerontol.* 2010; 4(4):224-228.

Roubenoff, R., Heymsfield, S. B., Kehayias, J. J., Cannon, J. G., Rosenberg, I. H. Standardization of nomenclature of body composition in weight loss. *Am J Clin Nutr.* 1997; 66:192-6.

Rodrigues, E. V., Valderramas, S. R., Rossetin, L. L., Gomes, A. R. S. Effects of Video Game Training on the Musculoskeletal Function of Older Adults: A Systematic Review and Meta-analysis. *Top Geriatr Rehabil.* 2014; 30(4):238-245.

Rogers, C. Presbyastasis: A multifactorial cause of balance problems in the elderly. *SA Fam Pract.* 2010; 52(5):431-434.

Rossi, L. P., Pereira, R., Brandalize, M., Gomes, A. R. S. The Effects of a Perturbation-Based Balance Training on the Reactive Neuromuscular Control in Community: Dwelling Older Women: A Randomized Controlled Trial. *Human Movement.* 2013; 14(3):238-246.

Ryan, J. G., Schertzer, J. D., Lynch, G. S. Cellular and molecular mechanisms underlying age-related skeletal muscle wasting and weakness. *Biogerontology,* 2008; 9:213-228.

Sakamoto, K., Nakamura, T., Hagino, H., Endo, N., Mori, S., Muto, Y. et al., Effects of unipedal standing balance exercise on the prevention of falls and hip fracture among clinically defined high-risk elderly individuals: A randomized controlled trial. *J Orthop Sci.* 2006; 5: 467-72.

Secchi, K. V., Morais, C. P., Cimatti, P. F., Tokars, E., Gomes, A. R. S. Efeito do alongamento e do exercício contra-resistido no músculo esquelético de rato. *Rev. bras. Fisioter.* 2008; 12(3):228-34.

Segev-Jacubovski, O., Herman, T., Yogev-Seligmann, G., Mirelman, A., Giladi, N., Hausdorff, J. M. The interplay between gait, falls and cognition: Can cognitive therapy reduce fall risk? *Expert Rev Neurother.* 2011; 11(7):1057-1075.

Shier, I. Does streching improve performance? A systematic and critical review of the literature. *Clin J Sport Med.* 2004; 14:267-273.

Singh, D. K. A., Rajaratnam, B. S., Palaniswamy, V., Raman, V. P., Bong, P. S., Pearson, H. Effects of balance-focused interactive games compared to therapeutic balance classes for older women. *Climacteric.* 2013; 16(1): 141-146.

Singh, D. K., Rajaratnam, B. S., Palaniswamy, V., Pearson, H., Raman, V. P., Bong, P. S. Participating in a virtual reality balance exercise program can reduce risk and fear of falls. *Maturitas.* 2012; 73(3):239-43.

Skelton, D. A., Greig, C. A., Davies, J. M., Young, A. Strength, power and related functional ability of healthy people aged 65-89 years. *Age Ageing.* 1994 Sep; 23(5):371-7.

Soucie, J. M., Wang, C., Forsyth, A., Funk, S., Denny, M., Roach, K. E. et al., Range of motion measurements: reference values and a database for comparison studies. *Haemophilia.* 2011;17(3):500-7.

Sperotto, F. M., Spinelli, R. B. *Avaliação nutricional em idosos independentes de uma instituição de longa permanência no Município de Erechim - RS.* Perspectiva. 2010 mar [citado em 11 nov 2010]; 34(125):105-116. Consulted in: http://www.uricer.edu.br/new/site/pdfs/perspectiva/125_78.pdf.

Stanziano, D. C., Roos, B. A., Perry, A. C., Lai, S., Signorile, J. F. The effects of an active-assisted stretching program on functional performance in elderly persons: A pilot study. *Clin Interv Aging.* 2009; 4: 115-20.

Stenroth, L., Peltonen, J., Cronin, N. J., Sipilä, S., Finni, T. Age related differences in Achilles tendon properties and triceps surae muscle architecture *in vivo. J Appl Physiol.* 2012; 113: 1537-1544.

Sturnieks, D. L., Tiedemann, A., Chapman, K., Munro, B., Murray, S. M., Lord, S. R. Physiological risk factors for falls in older people with lower limb arthritis. *J Rheumatol.* 2004; 31(11); 2272-2279.

Suetterlin, K. J., Sayer, A. A. Proprioception: Where are we now? A commentary on clinical assessment, changes across the life course, functional implications and future interventions. *Age Ageing.* 2014; 43: 313-318.

Szturm, T., Betker, A. L., Moussavi, Z., Desai, A., Goodman, V. Effects of an interactive computer game exercise regimen on balance impairment in frail community-dwelling older adults: A randomized controlled trial. *Phys Ther.* 2011; 91(10):1449-62.

Taylor, D. C., Dalton, J. D., Seaber, A. V., Garrett W. E. Viscoelastic properties of muscle-tendon units. The biomechanical effects of stretching. *Am J Sports Med.* 1990; 18: 300-9.

Teixeira, I. N. D. O. & Néri, A. L. *A fragilidade no envelhecimento: Fenômeno multidimensional, multideterminado e evolutivo.* In: Freitas EV, Py L, Cançado F., Doll J., Gorzoni M. L. Tratado de geriatria e geronlogia 2. ed. Rio de Janeiro: Guanabara Koogan: 2006, (115):1102-9.

Thompsom, L. Skeletal Muscle Adaptations with Age, Inactivity, and Therapeutic Exercise. *J Orthop & Sports Physic. Ther.* 2002; 32(2):44-57.

Toulotte, C., Toursel, C., Olivier, N. *Wii Fit®* training vs. Adapted Physical Activities: Which one is the most appropriate to improve the balance of independent senior subjects? A randomized controlled study. *Clin Rehabil.* 2012; 26(9):827-35.

Trappe, T. Influence of aging and long-term unloading on the structure and function of human skeletal muscle. *Appl Physiol Nutr Metab.* 2009; 34: 459-464.

Van Impe, A., Coxon, J. P., Goble, D. J., Doumas, M., Swinnen, S. P. White matter fractional anisotropy predicts balance performance in older adults. *Neurobiol Aging.* 2012; 33(9):1900-12.

Van Leeuwen, D. M., Ruiter, A. J., Nolte A. P., de Haan, A. *Preoperative Strength Training for Elderly Patients Awaiting Total Knee Arthroplasty.* 2014; 2014:462750. doi: 10.1155/2014/462750. Epub 2014.

Walston, J., Hadley, E. C., Ferruci, L., Guralnik, J. M., Newman, A. B., Studenski, S. A. et al., Research agenda for frailty in older adults: Toward a better understanding of physiology an etiology: Summary from the American Geriatrics Society/National Institute on Aging Research Conference on Frailty in Older Adults. *J Am Geriatr Soc.* 2006; 54(6): 991-1001.

Watt, J. R., Jackson, K., Franz, J. R., Dicharry, J., Evans, J., Kerrigan, D. C. Effect of a supervised hip flexor stretching program on gait in elderly individuals. *PMR.* 2011; 3(4):324-9.

Weppler, C. H., Magnusson, S. P. Increasing muscle extensibility: A matter of increasing length or modifying sensation. *Phys Ther,* 2010; 90(3):438-449.

Wu, T. Y., Chie, W. C., Yang, R. S., Liu, J. P., Kuo, K. L., Wong, W. K., Liaw, C. K. Factors Associated with Falls Among Community-Dwelling Older People in Taiwan. *Ann Acad Med.* 2013; 42(7): 320-327.

Zöllner A. M., Abilez O. J., Böl M., Kuhl E. Stretching skeletal muscle: Chronic muscle lengthening through sarcomerogenesis. *PLoS One*. 2012; 7(10):e45661.

Zotz, T. G. G., Loureiro, A. P. C., Valderramas, S. R., Gomes, A. R. S. *Stretching: An important strategy to prevent musculoskeletal aging: A systematic review and meta-analysis.* Topics in Geriatric Rehabilitation, 2014 DOI: 10.1097/TGR.0000000000000032 inpress.

Index

C

D

G

H

I

J

K

L

M

N

O

P

Q

R

S

T

U

V

W

Y